AF332972

IMMUNOLOGY OF BEHÇET'S DISEASE

Immunology of Behçet's disease

Edited by

MANFRED ZIERHUT
Department of Ophthalmology, University of Tübingen, Germany

and

SHIGEAKI OHNO
Department of Ophthalmology and Visual Sciences, Hokkaido University, Sapporo, Japan

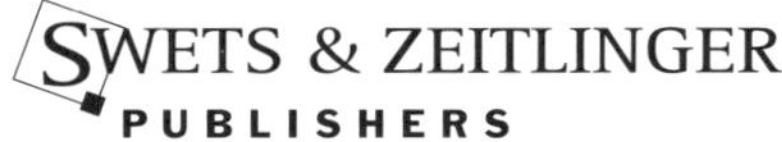

SWETS & ZEITLINGER
PUBLISHERS

LISSE　　　ABINGDON　　　EXTON (PA)　　　TOKYO

Library of Congress Cataloging-in-Publication Data

Applied for

Cover design: Studio Jan de Boer, Amsterdam
Typesetting: Martin Fischer, Tübingen
Printed in the Netherlands by Grafisch Produktiebedrijf Gorter bv, Steenwijk

Published by: Swets & Zeitlinger Publishers
www.szp.swets.nl

ISBN 90 265 1960 5

Contents

Contents

Foreword

Behçet´s Disease (BD) is one of the most-studied systemic disorders characterized by an occlusive vasculopathy of multiple organs. Various international meetings have established diagnostic criteria, so we now recognize most cases of BD and can start adequate treatment.

The etiology, and pathogenesis of BD are still unclear, but there is evidence for genetic, immunologic (probably autoimmunologic) and infectious factors in the onset and throughout the course of the disease.

This book highlights various aspects of BD. After an epidemiological overview and a discussion of the study of the frequency of diseases like BD, the clinical presentation of ocular and non-ocular symptoms of BD will be summarized. The immunopathological changes reflect a chronic vasculitis of arterioles, venules and capillaries.

BD seems to be a TH1-driven disease. So, the role of T-cells, but also of NK-T-cells and secreted cytokines, is covered. Also, neutrophil hyperfunction is a well-studied important characteristic of BD.

For years, herpes simplex virus, streptococcal or other infections have been under investigation as initiating antigens of BD. In particular, immune reactions against various microbial heat shock proteins could be an important etiological factor in BD.

The role of HLA-B51 as the major genetic factor has been known for over 20 years, but there seems to be other associations, possibly the transmembrane major histocompatibility complex (MHC) class I related gene A (MICA) allele A6. The peptide motif of HLA-B*5101 is well characterized and may likely help the possible elucidation of disease mechanisms.

Microsatellite mapping of the HLA-B*51 has shown that the pathogenic gene involved in the development of BD is pinpointed to HLA-B*51. Animal models like transgenic mice carrying the MHC class I related gene A (MICA) or B (MICB) may help to find the relative role of immune defects, infections and genetic factors.

Finally, the treatment of BD will be discussed in detail. It seems that the use of anti-TNF-alpha-antibodies, and also of interferon-alpha, has changed the prognosis of BD, which in previous years was regarded as being very bad due to occlusive vasculopathy of the retinal and the optic nerve vessels.

This book summarizes our knowledge regarding the most important factors that induce or trigger BD. We hope that it stimulates research in this field and helps to initiate new ideas.

MANFRED ZIERHUT
SHIGEAKI OHNO

CHRISTOS C. ZOUBOULIS

1. Epidemiology of Adamantiades-Behçet's Disease

ABSTRACT

Adamantiades-Behçet's disease is a universal disorder with varying prevalence, i.e. 80–370 pat/100,000 inhabitants in Turkey, 2–30 in the Asian continent and 0.1–7.5 in Europe and the USA. Certain ethnic groups are mainly affected. The prevalence of the disease seems to be strongly dependent on the geographic area of their residence. These data indicate environmental triggering of a genetically determined disorder. The disease usually occurs around the 3rd decade of life, however, early and late onsets (1–72 y) have been reported. Juvenile onset disease rates 7–44% in different ethnic groups; juvenile disease is less frequent (2–21%). Both genders are equally affected. Familial occurrence has been reported in 1–18% of patients, mostly Turks, Israeli and Koreans, and is increased in patients with juvenile disease. Oral aphthous ulcers represent the onset sign in the majority of patients worldwide (47–86%). Oral aphthous ulcers (92–100%), genital ulcerations (57–93%), skin lesions (38–99%), ocular lesions (29–100%) and arthropathy (16–84%) are the most frequent clinical features; sterile pustules (28–66%) and erythema nodosum (15–78%) are the most common skin lesions. The positivity of pathergy test varies widely in different populations (6–71%). HLA-B51 is associated with high relative risk for the disease in the Mediterranean Sea countries and Southern Asia. Diagnosis can be established 2–15 y after the onset of the disease. Male gender, early development of the disease in adults, and HLA-B51 positivity are markers of severe prognosis (mortality 0–6%).

KEYWORDS: Epidemiology, Adamantiades-Behçet's disease, Behçet's disease

INTRODUCTION

Adamantiades-Behçet's disease is a rather rare disorder with wide distribution but varying prevalence around the world. It occurs endemically in the Eastern Mediterranean and in Central and East Asian countries. The spread of these geographic areas along the old silk route and associated immunogenetic data support the hypothesis that the disease was carried over through the immigration of old nomadic tribes [1]. Transfer of genetic material or of an exogenous agent may have been responsible for the expansion of the disease.

PREVALENCE

The highest prevalence of the disease has been reported in Turks living in Anatolia (Northeastern Turkey) with 370 patients per 100,000 inhabitants [2], while the overall prevalence in Asia is 10- to 150-fold lower and in Europe and the U.S.A. more than 150-fold lower [2–17] (Table 1). Single or a few cases have been reported in all continents.

Interestingly, in areas with many ethnic populations, certain ethnic groups are mainly affected. In Taiwan, all 103 patients diagnosed between 1970 and 1988 were Chinese [18]. In Iran, Turks present a significantly higher prevalence than Caucasians and Semites, while no patient was found among Zoroastrians, who are isolated-living Caucasians [19]. In Kuwait, Kuwaiti bedouins are not affected by the disease and there is only a prevalence of 1.58 per 100,000 Kuwaitis which is similar to the involvement of non-Arab populations (1.35 per 100,000 inhabitants) and lower than 2.90 per 100,000 non-Kuwaiti Arabs [12]. In Berlin-West, Germany, the disease exhibited a prevalence of 20.75 per 100,000 inhabitants of Turkish origin compared to only 0.42 per 100,000 inhabitants of German origin in the year 1989 [5].

In populations with the same ethnic origin the prevalence of the disease seems to be strongly dependent on the longitude or the latitude of their residence. The prevalence in Turkish populations was calculated to decrease up to 18-fold by increasing distance from Eastern Turkey towards a western direction (Table 1). On the other hand, the prevalence of the disease in Japan was assessed to decrease up to 30-fold by moving from northern to southern Japan and to be annihilated in Japanese living in Hawaii [10] and in the U.S.A. [11]. A few patients of Japanese origin were found in Brazil [20]. These data indicate (an) environmental factor(s) which possibly trigger(s) the onset or the development of the disease in genetically determined populations.

Studies comparing epidemiological features of the disease over the time have found a throughout increasing prevalence, which may be due to the chronic character of the disease. In Japan, there were 7.0–8.5 patients per 100,000 inhabitants in the year 1972 [21], 8.3–10.0 patients per 100,000 inhabitants in the year 1984 [9] and 13.5 patients per 100,000 inhabitants in the year 1991 [9]. In Berlin-West, Germany, 0.65 patients per 100,000 inhabitants were detected in the year 1984, 1.68 patients per 100,000 inhabitants in the year 1989 and 2.26 patients per 100,000 inhabitants in the year 1994 [5]. In Rome, Italy, Adamantiades-Behçet's disease was found responsible for 3% of uveitis between 1968 and 1977, but for as much as 7.5% between 1978 and 1987 [22].

Table 1   Worldwide distribution of Adamantiades-Behçet's disease.

Population	Year	Prevalence per 100,000 inhabitants	
		Country	Region
ASIA			
Turkish			
Ordu region, Northeastern Anatolia [2]	1987		370
Ankara region [3]	1998		115
European part [4]	1981		80
Berlin-West, Germany [5]	1989		20.75
Saudi Arabian, Al Qassim region [6]	1997		20
Iranian [7]	1996	16.67	
Chinese [8]	1998	14.00	
Japanese [9]	1991	13.50	
Hokkaido region [9]	1991		30.50
Kyushu region [9]	1991		0.99
Hawaii [10]	1975		0
U.S.A. [11]	1979		0
Kuwait [12]	1986	2.10	
Kuwaitis [12]	1986		1.58
Non-Kuwaiti Arabs [12]	1986		2.90
Non-Arabs [12]	1986		1.35
Kuwaiti bedouins [12]	1986		0
AFRICA			
Egyptian, Alexandria region [13]	1997		7.60
EUROPE [5]			
Spaniard			
Northern Spain [14]	1998		7.50
Galicia [15]	2000		0.66
Italian	1988	2.50	
Germany, Berlin-West area	1994		2.26
German	1994		0.55
Portuguese	1993	1.53	
Swedish	1993	1.18	
British	1987	0.50	
Yorkshire region	1977		0.64
Scotland	1992		0.27
AMERICA			
U.S. American [16]	1979	0.12	
Olmsted County, MN [17]	1985		0.33
Hawaii [10]	1975	0	

INCIDENCE

Data on the incidence of the disease are rather sparing and ambiguous. In Japan, a country with well organized registration of patients with Adamantiades-Behçet's disease, 0.89 new cases per 100,000 inhabitants have been diagnosed in the year 1984 [9]. In 1990, 0.75 new cases per 100,000 inhabitants have been registered indicating the reaching of a plateau after a rapid increase of incidence since 1972. In Taiwan, the yearly number of patients who first visited six major medical centers from 1979 to 1983 was about 5, while about 14 patients per year presented for the first time from 1984 to 1988 [18].

AGE OF ONSET

The disease usually occurs around the third decade of life, an observation which is independent of the origin of the patients or their gender (Table 2). An average age of onset of 31.7 years was recorded in countries of East Asia, 26.5 years in Arab countries, 25.6 years in Turkey, 19.9 years in Israel, 25.9 years in Europe and 28.3 years in Americas. However, cases with early and late onset of the disease have also been reported and the age of onset ranges between the first months of life and 72 years.

The rate of patients with juvenile onset of the disease is varying among the several populations from 44.1% in Israel [34], 30.4% in the U.S.A. [40], 22.0% in Korea [24], 14.1% in Iran [47], 10.7% in patients of German origin [48], 7.6% in Italy [49] to 7.1% in Morocco [50]. Juvenile disease is less frequent, its prevalence was estimated in France to be 0.17 patients per 100,000 inhabitants [51]. Juvenile disease was reported in 20.8% of patients in Greece [52], 11.3% in Jordan [53], 8.6% in India [28], 6.1% in Turkey [54], 4.8% of patients with German origin [48], 4.3% of patients in Iran [47], 4.3% in U.S. American patients [40], 3.5% in Morocco [50], 2.3% in Tunisia [55] and 1.5% of patients in Japan [21].

SEX DISTRIBUTION

In contrast to old Japanese [56] and Turkish [57] reports of an androtropism, the male-to-female ratio drastically decreased in the last 20 years to currently reach an equal rate [9, 31, 58]. Similar observations were made in Israel [34, 59] and in Germany [5] (Fig. 1). Current epidemiological studies register an approximately equal male-to-female ratio in several populations (Table 2). An androtropism is still observed in Arab countries, while gynaecotropism is evident in some northern European countries and in the U.S.A.

Japanese studies has shown a real increase in female patients which is associated with a trend towards a mild clinical course of the disease [9].

Table 2   Demographic data on Adamantiades-Behçet's disease in a worldwide comparison.

Country	Number of patients	Age of onset, y		Male : Female ratio
		average	range (SD)	
ASIA				
Japan [9]	1139	35.7		1.07 : 1
Korea [23]	1155	28.8	7–71	0.63 : 1
China [24]	328	27.9	4–58	0.69 : 1
Taiwan [18, 25]	156		10–50	2.47 : 1
Philippines [26]	9			2.00 : 1
Singapore [27]	34	37		0.55 : 1
India [28]	58	33.1	10–64	1.76 : 1
Iran [7]	3153	26.2	(± 9.7)	1.13 : 1
Iraq [29]	60	29.4		3.00 : 1
Saudi Arabia [30]	119	22.9	13–51	3.40 : 1
Kuwait [12]	29			3.10 : 1
Turkey [31]	2147	25.6		1.03 : 1
Lebanon [32]	32	22.0	3–45	1.50 : 1
Jordan [33]	150	25.2	(± 9.4)	3.40 : 1
Israel [34]	59	19.9	2–54	0.79 : 1
AFRICA				
Egypt [13]	274	26.2	(± 9.9)	5.37 : 1
Tunisia [35]	702	28.9	(± 9.9)	3.00 : 1
Morocco [36]	673	31.7	5–60	2.54 : 1
South Africa [37]	5			0.67 : 1
EUROPE [5]				
Russia	25	24.7	(±12.9)	0.56 : 1
Czech Republic [38]	9			2.00 : 1
Sweden	5	33.0	19–48	0.67 : 1
Scotland	15			0.36 : 1
England	53	24.7	10–61	0.96 : 1
Ireland	24	20.8	(± 7.5)	1.40 : 1
Germany*	96	24.5	0–72	1.00 : 1
Portugal	241	25.7	(±11.1)	1.01 : 1
Spain*	47	26.9	12–48	1.35 : 1
France	126	28.5	2–64	1.57 : 1
Italy	155	25.0	5–53	2.44 : 1
Yugoslavia [39]	21			1.33 : 1
Greece	63	29.0	5–67	1.42 : 1
AMERICA				
U.S.A. [40, 41]	131	25.6	5–49	0.42 : 1
Brazil [20, 42–44]	197	30.2	9–61	0.91 : 1
Chile [45]	5			4.00 : 1
OCEANIA				
Australia [46]	12			2.00 : 1

* modified to include current data

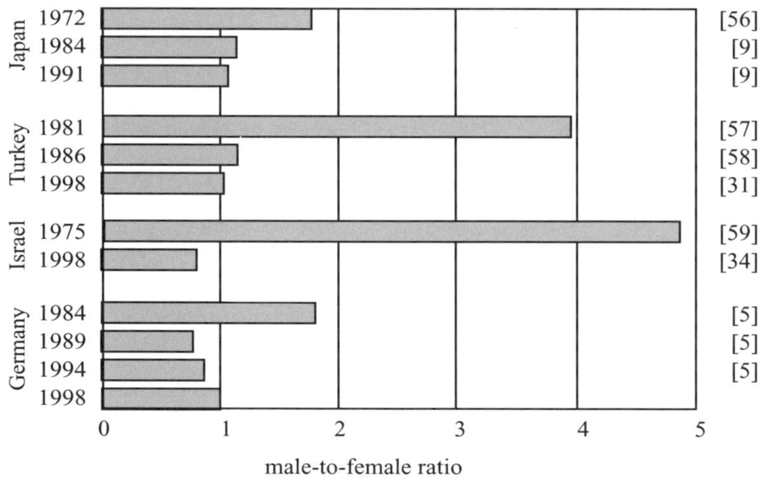

Figure 1 Development of male-to female ratio over time.

FAMILIAL OCCURRENCE

Familial occurrence is one of the major epidemiological features of Adamantiades-Behçet's disease. Interestingly, familial occurrence is more frequent in families with Korean (15.4%) than Japanese or Chinese (2.2–2.6%) origin (p<0.001, χ^2 test). Also patients with Arab, Israeli or Turkish origin presented higher frequencies of familial cases (2.0–18.2%) than European patients (0–4.5%; p<0.001, χ^2 test) (Table 3).

In juvenile patients there is a higher frequency of familial occurrence than in adults, namely 16% vs. 2% in Morocco [71], 18% vs. 2% in France [51] and 25% vs. 8% in Germany [48]. Recently, genetic anticipation in the form of earlier disease onset in children compared to their parents has been identified corroborating the findings of higher frequency of familial cases in juveniles than in adults and the possibility of a genetic predisposition in Adamantiades-Behçet's disease [72].

ONSET MANIFESTATIONS

Oral aphthous ulcers represent the onset feature of the disease in the majority of the patients worldwide (47–86%) (Table 4). Genital ulcerations (0–18%), skin lesions (0–27%) – especially erythema nodosum (0–19%) –, ocular lesions (0–35%), arthropathy (0–24%), neurological features (0–12%) and vascular involvement (0–3%) can also occur as onset lesions. The high frequencies of oral aphthous ulcers, genital ulcerations, skin and ocular lesions as onset signs confirm the importance of these clinical features for diagnosis. Highly recurrent oral aphthosis, the most frequent onset sign, is a warning signal for Adamantiades Behçet's disease. Fifty-two per cent of 67 prospectively evaluated patients with recurrent oral aphthosis (in average 10 recurrences per year) in Korea developed Adamantiades-Behçet's disease in 8 years after

                    Christos C. Zouboulis

Table 3 Familial occurrence of Adamantiades-Behçet's disease.

Population	number of patients	rate (%)
ASIA		
Turkish		
Turkey [60]	170	18.2
Germany [5]*	101	15.5
Israeli [61]	38	13.2
Korean [23]	178	15.4
Indian [28]	58	13.8
Saudi-Arabs [30]	119	7.5
Lebanese [32]	32	6.3
Iranian [62]	1242	5.5
Chinese [63]		2.6
Japanese [64, 73]	223	2.2
AFRICA		
Egyptian [13]	274	10.7
Moroccan [36]	673	5.6
Tunisian		
North Tunisia [35]	702	2.0
South Tunisia [65]	26	11.9
EUROPE		
Spaniard [15, 66]	38	5.3
English [67]	33	3.6
German [5]*	96	3.2
Portuguese [68]	154	2.6
Italian [22, 69]	177	1.3
Greek [70]	64	1.3

* modified to include current data

development of oral aphthous ulcers [74]. Although it is also a frequent feature, arthropathy is unspecific and, therefore, does not support diagnosis if it occurs as onset sign of the disease.

CLINICAL FINDINGS

Oral aphthous ulcers (92–100%), genital ulcerations (57–93%), skin lesions (38–99%), ocular lesions (29–100%) and arthropathy (16–84%) are the most frequent features of the disease worldwide (Table 5). Sterile pustules (28–66%) and erythema nodosum (15–78%) are the most frequent skin lesions. A positive pathergy test is

Table 4   Onset manifestations of Adamantiades-Behçet's disease (%).

Nationality	Japan [73]	Korea [23]	China [63]	Iraq [29]	Iran [7]	Turkey [31]	Israel [34]	Egypt [13]	Europe [5][a]	Brazil [44]	Australia [46]
Number of patients	85	1155	328[b]	60	3153	2147	59	274[c]	353	81	12
Oral aphthous ulcers	52	79	56	47	77	86	60	60	58–78	47	75
Genital ulcerations	4	7	10	10	10[d]	7	17	18	2–7	–	8
Skin lesions	19	11	27	12		5	11	–	7–26	12	8
Folliculitis/sterile pustules			5			2	–		1		
Erythema nodosum			19			3	11		8–14		8
Superf. thrombophlebitis			–			1	–		1–5		
Ocular lesions	21	3	4	13	12	1	–	23	1–18	35	25
Arthropathy	4	–	–	13	7	1	13	6	5–24	6	
Neurological features	–	–	–	2		–	–	3	0–9	12	
Vascular involvement	–	–	–	2		–	2	3	–	–	
Other manifestations				2	9[e]						

[a] Europe [5]: England, n=39; France, n=133; Germany, n=96 (modified to include current data); Greece, n=63; Spain, n=38;
[b] Multiple site onset lesions in 5%;
[c] Multiple site onset lesions in 16%;
[d] Mostly accompanied by oral aphthosis;
[e] Mostly skin manifestations.

Table 5   Clinical findings of Adamantiades-Behçet's disease (%).

Nationality	Japan	Korea	Taiwan	China	India	Iraq	Iran	Kuwait	Saudi-Arabia	Turkey	Lebanon	Jordan	Israel	Egypt	Tunisia	Morocco	Europe[a]	U.S.A.	Brasil
	[9]	[23]	[18]	[24]	[28]	[29]	[7]	[12]	[30]	[31]	[32]	[33]	[34]	[13]	[35]	[36]	[5][a]	[40, 41]	[20, 42–44]
Number of patients	3316	1155	103	328	58	60	3153	103	119	2147	32	150	59	274	702	601	714	131	197
Oral aphthous ulcers	98	98	97	100	90	97	96	100	100	100	97	100	100	92	99	100	98–100	99	99
Genital ulcerations	73	57	61	84	78	83	64	93	87	88	78	85	68	76	80	84	65–91	86	68
Skin lesions	87	61	75	99	64	75	74	76	57	54	38	90	86	39			66–84	98	66
Folliculitis/ sterile pustules		36		40		48	66		53	54	28				55	61	41–49	48	52
Erythema nodosum		55		64	47	55	23		47	47	19	41			20	15	25–78	37	36
Ulcerations		2		1						16						5	0–13	22	8
Superf. thrombophlebitis		3		4	24				13	11	6	7					4–29		
Positive pathergy test	44			66	9	71	61	34	18	57	71	55	46	70	50	68	12–52	33	6
Ocular lesions	69	29	100	40	43	48	59	69	56	29	59	46	49	76	50	67	35–69[d]	37	79
Arthropathy	57	24	61	58	71	48	41	69	37	16	75	53	83	56	30	64	33–84	34	61
Neurological features	11	6	3	2	4	2	4	14	44	2	19	28	15	26	17	14	11–48	18	8
Vascular involvement	9		2	8	10	17	9	34	34	17	6	29	29	23[c]	17	21	10–37	14	17
Gastrointestinal features	16	4	15	9	5	10	9	21	4	3	13	19		10	1	13	5–60	–	6
Prostatitis–Epididymitis[b]	6		6	6	–	22	11		4		3	28		16	4		2–44	–	17
Chest disease		3	+	–		1	7	16	1	3	9			1	–	2	0–17	–	3
Kidney involvement		5	–	2		–	7	6	+		5			–	1	0–10	–	..–	
Cardiac disease		–	3	–		1	–	–	+		2			–	3	0–7	–	4	

[a] Europe: Czech Republic, n=9 [38]; England, n=46; France, n=133; Germany, n=96 (modified to include current data); Greece, n=63; Italy, n=141; Portugal, n=142; Russia, n=25; Spain, n=38; Yugoslavia, n=21 [39];
[b] Male;
[c] including cardiac disease;
[d] Czech and Italian patients were excepted;
+ Present lesions in less than 0.5% of patients.

reported in 6–71% of the different patients groups. A comparison of the frequencies of clinical features among patients of different ethnic origin revealed lower rates of positive pathergy test in patients in Europe, the U.S.A. and Brazil (32%) than in patients in the rest of the world (54%, p<0.001, χ^2 test) and higher rates of arthropathy in Europeans, U.S. Americans and Brazilian (62%) than in the latter group (41%; p<0.001, χ^2 test). Gastrointestinal features were assessed to be more frequent in Japanese and Europeans (16%) than in Korean and Turkish patients (3%, p<0.001, χ^2 test). A comparison concerning the rates of ocular lesions in south-eastern European patients (Italian and Greek) and south-western as well as northern European patients has detected significantly higher rates in the former group [5].

ASSOCIATION OF HLA-B51 WITH THE DISEASE

HLA-B51 is significantly associated with Adamantiades-Behçet's disease [1]. It is surprising, however, that none of the functional correlates of the disease appear to be restricted by HLA-B51. Current evidence is shifting towards the view that HLA-B51 is not involved directly in the etiology of the disease [75] but might be closely linked to disease-related gene(s) [76]. On the other hand, HLA-B51 was found to be a marker for unfavorable prognosis, especially an earlier development of the disease, ocular lesions and vessel involvement [5]. HLA-B5 positive individuals of German origin as well as from other northern European countries were detected to present a lower relative risk to develop the disease compared to southern Europeans, especially patients from south-eastern European countries [5]. It is interesting that the relative risk of HLA-B51 individuals to develop the disease does not follow the distribution of the HLA-B51 allele around the world (Table 6); it is increased in a small geographic area which well correlates with the major antic trade routes [101] (Fig. 2).

COURSE AND PROGNOSIS

Adamantiades-Behçet's disease is usually diagnosed with a delay of several years after the appearance of the onset sign, i.e. after 1 year in Israel [34], 2.1 years in Iraq [29], 3 years in Germany [5], 4.7 years in India [28], 5.1 years in Spain [14], 6.1 years in Turkey [31], 6.4 years in Saudi Arabia [30], 6.4 years in Korea [102], 7.8 years in Russia [103], 8 years in the U.S.A. [40, 104], 5–15 years in Japan [105]. The disease exhibits a potentially severe course with mortality rates of 0 to 6.3%, mostly involving male patients (Table 7). The real increase of female cases in Japan is associated with a decrease of the mortality rate, namely from 1% in 1972 to 0.4% in 1991 [9]. Central nervous system, pulmonary as well as large vessel involvement and bowel perforation are the major life-threatening manifestations. On the other hand, blindness and the consequences of central nervous system involvement are the most disabling features. There is evidence that a lethal outcome is often due to delayed diagnosis and treatment. In addition to HLA-B51 positivity, male gender [5] and early development of systemic features [110] have been detected to be markers of severe prognosis, while juvenile onset does not predict unfavorable prognosis [34, 48, 110]. Spontaneous

Table 6 Frequency of HLA-B51 antigen in patient groups and relative risk (RR) for Adamantiades-Behçet's disease.

Country	Patients n	Patients HLA-B51+ in%	Controls n	Controls HLA-B51+ in%	RR
ASIA					
Japan [76]	91	57	140	14	7.9
Korea [77]	52	44	42	17	4.0
Taiwan [78]	51	51	128	11	8.5
China [79]	120	56	100	12	9.3
India [28, 80]	31	32	400		
Iraq [29]	52	62	175	29	3.9
Iran [81]		53		33	2.3
Turkey [5, 57, 82–84]	520	77	1106	26	9.2
Saudi Arabia [30]	85	72		26	9.0
Jordan [33]	68	74	43	23	9.2
Israel [34, 61, 85, 86]	126	75	790	21	11.5
AFRICA					
Egypt [87]	84	58	200	7	20.1
Tunisia [65, 88]	55	62	80	24	5.2
EUROPE [5]					
Russia	19	37	150	15	3.2
Great Britain	107	25	2032	9	3.3
Ireland	24	25	96	3	6.3
Germany*	70	37	1415	14	3.6
Switzerland	8	38		17	3.0
Portugal [89–91]	318	53	135	24	3.6
Spain [14, 66, 92]	100	42	452	21	2.7
France	105	51	591	13	6.7
Italy	57	75	304	22	10.9
Greece [93–97]	170	79	670	28	9.7
AMERICA					
U.S.A. [98, 99]	32	13	523	10	1.3
Mexico [100]	10	70	105	31	5.1

* modified to include current data

remissions of certain or of all manifestations or have been observed in a part of the patients several years after the onset of the disease [22, 24, 28, 63, 105].

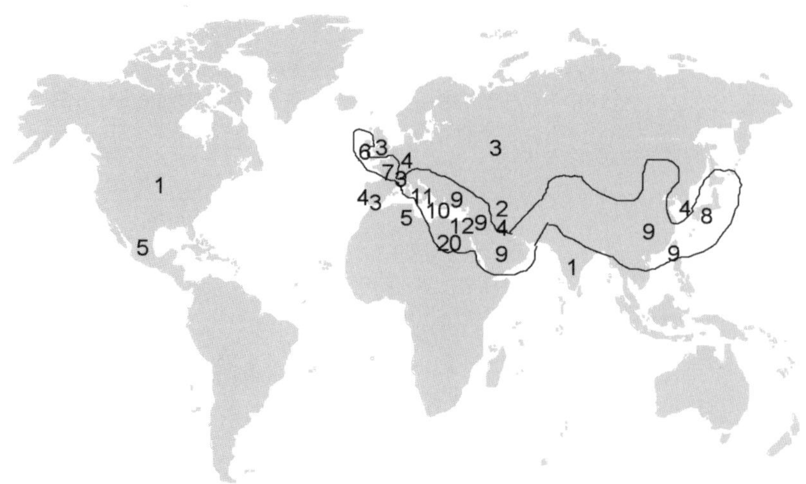

Figure 2 Worldwide relative risk for the development of Adamantiades-Behçet's disease in several countries.

Table 7 Mortality in Adamantiades-Behçet's disease

Country	Number of patients	Lethal outcome n=	%	Male	Female	Duration of follow-up (years)
England [106]	32	2	6.25			
Turkey [107]	120	6	5.00	6	–	10
France [108]	60	3	5.00			3 (1–12)
Germany [5]*	96	4	4.17	2	2	1–20
Spain [14]	30	1	3.33			
Italy [22]	141	4	2.84	4	–	>10
Portugal [68]	156	4	2.56	3	1	>10 (up to 21)
Saudi Arabia [30]	119	3	2.52			
Japan [9]	3316		0.40			
Korea [109]	2200	7	0.003	6	1	6.5
Greece [70]	64	–	0			
India [28]	58	–	0			4

* modified to include current data

CONCLUSION

Adamantiades-Behçet's disease is a rare, genetically determined, universal disorder whose presentation is probably associated with environmental triggering. The exact etiology remains unknown. The disease usually occurs around the 3rd decade of life with both genders being equally affected. Oral aphthous ulcers represent the onset sign

Christos C. Zouboulis

in the majority of patients worldwide, whereas oral aphthous ulcers, genital ulcerations, skin lesions, ocular lesions and arthropathy are the most frequent clinical features. Male gender, early development of the disease in adults, and HLA-B51 positivity are markers of severe prognosis.

REFERENCES

1. Ohno S, Ohguchi M, Hirose S, Matsuda H, Wakisaka A, Aizawa M. *Arch Ophthalmol* 100: 1455–8, 1982.
2. Yurdakul S, Günaydin I, Tüzün Y et al. *J Rheumatol* 15: 820–2, 1988.
3. Idil A, Gürler A, Boyvat A et al. in *8th International Congress on Behçet's Disease. Program and Abstracts*, Olivieri I, Salvarani C, Cantini F (eds.) p. 99, Prex, Milano, 1998.
4. Demirhindi O, Yazici H, Binyildiz P. *Cerrahp Tip Fak Derg* 12: 509–14, 1981.
5. Zouboulis ChC, Kötter I, Djawari D et al. *Yonsei Med J* 38: 411–22, 1997.
6. Al-Dalaan A, AlBallaa S, AlSukait M, Mousa M, Bahabri S, Biyari T. in *Behçet's disease*, Hamza M (ed.) pp. 170–2, Pub Adhoua, Tunis, 1997.
7. Shahram F, Davatchi F, Akbarian M, Gharibdoost F, Nadji A, Jamshidi AR. in *Behçet's disease*, Hamza M (ed.) pp. 165–9, Pub Adhoua, Tunis, 1997.
8. Davatchi F. in *8th International Congress on Behçet's Disease. Program and Abstracts*, Olivieri I, Salvarani C, Cantini F (eds.) p. 42, Prex, Milano, 1998.
9. Nakae K, Masaki F, Hashimoto T, Inaba G, Mochizuki M, Sakane T. in *Behçet's disease. International Congress Series 1037*, Wechsler B, Godeau P (eds.) pp. 145–51, Excerpta Medica, Amsterdam, 1993.
10. Hirohata T, Kuratsune M, Nomura A, Jimi S. *Hawaii Med J* 34: 244–6, 1975.
11. Ohno S, Char DH, Kimura SJ, O'Connor GR. *Jpn J Ophthalmol* 23: 126–31, 1979.
12. Mousa AR, Marafie AA, Rifai KM, Dajani AI, Mukhter MM. *Scand J Rheumatol* 15: 310–32, 1986.
13. Assaad-Khalil SH, Kamel FA, Ismail EA. in *Behçet's disease*, Hamza M (ed.) pp. 173–6, Pub Adhoua, Tunis, 1997.
14. Sanchez Burson J, Grandal Y, Mendoza M, Montero R, Rejón E, Marenco JL. in *8th International Congress on Behçet's Disease. Program and Abstracts*, Olivieri I, Salvarani C, Cantini F (eds.) p. 102, Prex, Milano, 1998.
15. González-Gay MA, García-Porrúa C, Brañas F, López-Lázaro L, Olivieri I. *J Rheumatol* 27: 703–7, 2000.
16. Chamberlain MA. in *Proceedings of a conference sponsored by the Royal Society of Medicine. February 1979*, pp. 213–22, Academic Press, London, 1979.
17. O'Duffy JD. *J Rheumatol* 5: 229–33, 1980.
18. Chung YM, Yeh TS, Sheu MM et al. *J Formos Med Assoc* 89: 413–7, 1990.
19. Davatchi F, Shahram F, Chams C et al. in *8th International Congress on Behçet's Disease. Program and Abstracts*, Olivieri I, Salvarani C, Cantini F (eds.) pp. 96–97, Prex, Milano, 1998.
20. Barra C, Belfort R Jr, Abreu MT, Kim MK, Martins MC, Petrilli AMN. *Jpn J Ophthalmol* 35: 339–46, 1991.
21. Maeda K, Nakae K. *Asian Med J* 2: 568–82, 1977.
22. Pivetti-Pezzi P. in *Ophthalmology Today*, Ferraz de Oliveira LN (ed.), pp. 81–93, Elsevier, New York, 1988.
23. Bang D, Yoon KH, Chung HG, Choi EH, Lee E-S, Lee S. *Yonsei Med J* 38: 428–36, 1977.
24. Cho MY, Lee SH, Bang D, Lee S. *Korean J Dermatol* 26: 320–9, 1988.

25. Chun SI, Su WPD, Lee S. *J Dermatol* 17:333–41, 1990.

26. Arroyo CG, Voctorio Navarra ST, Torralba TP. *Philippine J Intern Med* 31: 305–15, 1993.

27. Tan E, Chua SH, Lim JTE. *Ann Acad Med Singapore* 28: 440–4, 1999.

28. Pande I, Uppal SS, Kailash S, Kumar A, Malaviya AN. *Br J Rheumatol* 34: 825–30, 1995.

29. Al-Rawi ZS, Sharquie KE, Khalifa SJ, Al-Hadithi FM, Munir JJ. *Ann Rheum Dis* 45: 987–90, 1986.

30. Al-Dalaan A, Al Balaa SR, El Ramahi K et al. *J Rheumatol* 21: 658–61, 1994.

31. Gürler A, Boyvat A, Türsen Ü. *Yonsei Med J* 38: 423–7, 1997.

32. Bitar E, Ghayad E, Ghoussoub Kh. *Rev Rhum* 53: 621–4, 1986.

33. Madanat W, Fayyad F, Zureikat H et al. in *8th International Congress on Behçet's Disease. Program and Abstracts*, Olivieri I, Salvarani C, Cantini F (eds.) p. 255, Prex, Milano, 1998.

34. Krause I, Uziel Y, Guedj D et al. *J Rheumatol* 25: 1566–9, 1998.

35. Hamza M, Meddeb S. *Rev Rhum (Engl Ed)* 63: 538, 1996.

36. Benamour S, Chaoui L, Zeroual B et al. in *8th International Congress on Behçet's Disease. Program and Abstracts*, Olivieri I, Salvarani C, Cantini F (eds.) p. 232, Prex, Milano, 1998.

37. Jacyl WK. *J Am Acad Dermatol* 30: 869–73, 1994.

38. Rihová E, Havliková M, Michalová K, Rothová Z, Poch T. *Cs Oftal* 5: 298–304, 1997.

39. Mitrovic D, Popovic M, Pavlica L et al. *Vojnosanitetski Pregled* 54: 321–5, 1997.

40. Mangelsdorf HC, White WL, Jorizzo JL. *J Am Acad Dermatol* 34: 745–50, 1996.

41. Balabanova M, Calamia KT, O'Duffy JD. in *8th International Congress on Behçet's Disease. Program and Abstracts*, Olivieri I, Salvarani C, Cantini F (eds.) p. 118, Prex, Milano, 1998.

42. Rocha Lacerda R. in *Behçet's disease. International Congress Series 1037*, Wechsler B, Godeau P (eds.) pp. 185–8, Excerpta Medica, Amsterdam, 1993.

43. Scherrer MA, Vitral N, Orefice F. in *Behçet's disease. International Congress Series 1037*, Wechsler B, Godeau P (eds.) pp. 181–4, Excerpta Medica, Amsterdam, 1993.

44. Montenegro V, de Abreu AC, Schaimberg C, Gonçalves CR. in *8th International Congress on Behçet's Disease. Program and Abstracts*, Olivieri I, Salvarani C, Cantini F (eds.) p. 256, Prex, Milano, 1998.

45. Esguep AS, Quinteros IO. *J Oral Med* 42: 25–29, 1987.

46. Wakefield D, McCluskey P. *Aust N Z J Ophthalmol* 18: 129–35, 1990.

47. Shahram F, Shafaie N, Davatchi F, Nadji A, Akbarian M, Jamshidi A. in *8th International Congress on Behçet's Disease. Program and Abstracts*, Olivieri I, Salvarani C, Cantini F (eds.) p. 180, Prex, Milano, 1998.

48. Treudler R, Orfanos CE, Zouboulis ChC. *Dermatology* 199: 15–19, 1999.

49. Pivetti Pezzi P, Accorinti M, Abdulaziz MA, La Cava M, Torella M, Riso D. *Jpn J Ophthalmol* 39: 309–14, 1995.

50. Benamour S, Tak-Tak T, Moudatir A et al. in *8th International Congress on Behçet's Disease. Program and Abstracts*, Olivieri I, Salvarani C, Cantini F (eds.) p. 176, Prex, Milano, 1998.

51. Koné-Paut I, Bernard JL. *Arch Fr Pediatr* 50: 561–3, 1993.

52. Kaklamani VG, Vaiopoulos G, Markomichelakis N, Palimeris G, Markaki J, Kaklamanis Ph. in *8th International Congress on Behçet's Disease. Program and Abstracts*, Olivieri I, Salvarani C, Cantini F (eds.) p. 238, Prex, Milano, 1998.

53. Madanat W, Fayyad F, Zureikat H. in *8th International Congress on Behçet's Disease. Program and Abstracts*, Olivieri I, Salvarani C, Cantini F (eds.) p. 178, Prex, Milano, 1998.

54. Gürler A, Erdi H, Boyvat A. in *Behçet's disease*, Hamza M (ed.) pp. 139–42, Pub Adhoua, Tunis, 1997.

55. Hamza M. in *Behçet's disease. International Congress Series 1037*, Wechsler B, Godeau P (eds.) pp. 377–80, Excerpta Medica, Amsterdam, 1993.

                                                                 Christos C. Zouboulis

56. Yamamoto S, Toyokawa H, Matsubara J et al. *Jpn J Ophthalmol* 18: 282–90, 1974.

57. Müftüoglu AÜ, Yazici H, Yurdakul S et al. *Tissue Antigens* 17: 226–30, 1981.

58. Saylan T, Özarmagan G, Azizlerli G, Övül C, Öke N. *Zbl Hautkr* 61: 1120–2, 1986.

59. Chajek T, Fainaru M. Behçet's disease. *Medicine (Baltimore)* 54: 179–96, 1975.

60. Gül A, Inanç M, Öcal L, Aral O, Koniçe M. in *8th International Congress on Behçet's Disease. Program and Abstracts*, Olivieri I, Salvarani C, Cantini F (eds.) p. 98, Prex, Milano, 1998.

61. Arber N, Klein T, Meiner Z, Pras E, Weinberger A. *Ann Rheum Dis* 50: 351–3, 1991.

62. Shahram F, Chams C, Davatchi F, Nadji A, Akbarian, Jamshidi A. in *8th International Congress on Behçet's Disease. Program and Abstracts*, Olivieri I, Salvarani C, Cantini F (eds.) p. 103, Prex, Milano, 1998.

63. Hui-li S, Zheng-ji H. in *Behçet's disease. International Congress Series 1037*, Wechsler B, Godeau P (eds.) pp. 325–30, Excerpta Medica, Amsterdam, 1993.

64. Aoki K, Ohno S, Ohguchi M, Sugiura S. *Jpn J Clin Ophthalmol* 22: 72–5, 1978.

65. Makni H, Kolsi R, Kolsi S et al. in *Behçet's disease*, Hamza M (ed.) pp. 151–4, Pub Adhoua, Tunis, 1997.

66. Fernández Miranda C, Palacio Pérez-Medel A, Martínez-Martín P, Montalbán Pallarés MA, Domínguez Ortega L, Ramírez Díaz-Bernando J. *Rev Esp Reumatol* 10: 37–43, 1983.

67. Mason RM, Barnes CG. *Ann Rheum Dis* 28: 95–103, 1969.

68. de Souza-Ramalho P, D'Almeida MF, Freitas JP, Pinto J. *Acta Medica Portug* 4: 79–82, 1991.

69. Sensi A, Baricordi OR. *Br J Dermatol* 114: 748, 1986.

70. Kaklamani V, Vaiopoulos G, Kaklamanis Ph. *Sem Arthritis Rheum* 27: 197–217, 1998.

71. Benamour S, Tak-Tak MT, Rafik M, Anraoui A. in *Behçet's disease*, Hamza M (ed.) pp. 134–8, Pub Adhoua, Tunis, 1997.

72. Fresko I, Soy M, Hamuryudan V et al. *Ann Rheum Dis* 57: 45–8, 1998.

73. Oshima Y, Shimizu T, Yokohari R et al. *Ann Rheum Dis* 22: 36–45, 1963.

74. Bang D, Hur W, Lee E-S, Lee S. *J Dermatol* 22: 926–9, 1995.

75. Goto K, Mizuki N, Ohno S. in *Behçet's disease*, Hamza M (ed.) pp. 102–5, Pub Adhoua, Tunis, 1997.

76. Mizuki N, Inoko H, Mizuki N et al. *Invest Ophthalmol Vis Sci* 33: 3332–40, 1992.

77. Lee S, Koh YJ, Kim DH et al. *Yonsei Med J* 29: 259–62, 1988.

78. Chung Y-M, Tsai S-T, Liao F, Liu J-H. *Tissue Antigens* 30: 68–72, 1987.

79. Mineshita S, Tian D, Wang L-M et al. *Intern Med* 31: 1073–5, 1992.

80. Mehra NK, Taneja V, Kailash S, Raizada N, Vaidya MC. *Tissue Antigens* 27: 64–74, 1986.

81. Gharibdoost F, Davatchi F, Shahram F et al. in *Behçet's disease. International Congress Series 1037*, Wechsler B, Godeau P (eds.) pp. 153–8, Excerpta Medica, Amsterdam, 1993.

82. Azizlerli G, Aksungur VL, Sarica R, Akyol E, Övül C. *Dermatology* 188: 293–5, 1994.

83. Ersoy F, Berkel AI, Firat T, Kazokoglu H. *Arch Dermatol* 113: 1720–1, 1977.

84. Alpsoy E, Yilmaz E, Coskun M, Savas A, Yegin O. *J Dermatol* 25: 158–62, 1998.

85. Brautbar C, Chajek T, Ben-Tunia S, Lamm L, Cohen T. *Tissue Antigens* 11: 113–20, 1978.

86. Haim S, Gideoni O, Barzilai A. *Acta Dermatol Venereol (Stockh)* 57: 243–5, 1977.

87. Assaad-Khalil SH. in *Behçet's disease. Basic and clinical aspects,* O'Duffy JD, Kokmen E (eds.), pp. 269–77, Marcel Dekker, New York, 1991.

88. Hamza M, Ben Ayed HB, Sohier R, Betuel H. *Nouv Presse Med* 7: 3263, 1978.

89. Crespo J. *Rev Rhumatisme (engl ed)* 63: 538, 1996.

90. de Jesus H, Marques A, Rosa M, de Costa T, Queiroz MV. in *Behçet's disease*, Hamza M (ed.) pp. 204–5, Pub Adhoua, Tunis, 1997.

91. Vaz Patto J, Figueirinhas J, Parente M et al. in *Behçet's disease*, Hamza M (ed.) pp. 109–10, Pub Adhoua, Tunis, 1997.

92. González-Escribano MF, Rodríguez MR, Walter K, Sanchez-Roman J, García-Lozano JR, Núñez-Roldán A. *Tissue Antigens* 52: 78–80, 1998.

93. Psilas K, Polymenidis Z, Georgiades G. *J Fr Ophtalmol* 2: 701–4, 1979.

94. Palimeris G, Koliopoulos J, Theodossiadis G, Roussos J, Tsimbidas P. *Trans Ophthalmol Soc* UK 100: 527–30, 1980.

95. Zervas J, Vayopoulos G, Sakellaropoulos N, Kaklamanis Ph, Fessas Ph. *Clin Exp Rheumatol* 6: 277–80, 1988.

96. Messini H, Spyropoulou M, Papademitropoulos M et al. in *Behçet's disease*, Hamza M (ed.) pp. 106–8, Pub Adhoua, Tunis, 1997.

97. Koumantaki Y, Stavropoulos C, Spyropoulou M et al. *Hum Immunol* 59: 250–5, 1998.

98. O'Duffy JD, Taswell HF, Elverback LR. *J Rheumatol* 3: 1–3, 1978.

99. Ohno S, Char DH, Kimura SJ, O'Connor GR. *Jpn J Ophthalmol* 22: 58–61, 1978.

100. Lavalle C, Alarcon-Segovia D, Del Guidice-Knipping JA, Fraga A. *J Rheumatol* 8: 325–327, 1981.

101. Chapoutot-Remadi M. in *Behçet's disease*, Hamza M (ed.) pp. 22–9, Pub Adhoua, Tunis, 1997.

102. Kim HJ, Bang D, Lee SH et al. *Yonsei Med J* 29: 102–8, 1988.

103. Alekberova Z, Madanat W, Prokaeva T, Yermakova N, Poljanskaja I. in *Behçet's disease. International Congress Series 1037*, Wechsler B, Godeau P (eds.) pp. 171–4, Excerpta Medica, Amsterdam, 1993.

104. O'Duffy JD, Carney JA, Deodhar S. *Ann Intern Med* 75: 561–70, 1971.

105. Tanaka C, Haramoto S, Matsuda T et al. in *Behçet's disease*, Hamza M (ed.) pp. 217–8, Pub Adhoua, Tunis, 1997.

106. Chamberlain MA. *Ann Rheum Dis* 36: 491–9, 1977.

107. Yazici H, Basaran G, Hamuryudan V et al. *Br J Rheumatol* 35: 139–41, 1996.

108. Wechsler B, Piette JC, Conard J, Huong Du LT, Bletry O, Godeau P. *Presse Med* 16: 661–4, 1987.

109. Park KD, Bang D, Lee ES, Lee SH, Lee S. *J Korean Med Sci* 8: 241–5, 1993.

110. Saryca R, Azizlerli G, Köse A et al. in *Behçet's disease*, Hamza M (ed.) pp. 157–9, Pub Adhoua, Tunis, 1997.

Christos C. Zouboulis

HASAN YAZICI

2. A Proposal to Study the Frequency of Rare Diseases

ABSTRACT

We have recently proposed a method to determine an upper boundary for "zero" observations among a population of "n" individuals. Using the binomial distribution model, the upper limit of "n" was formulated to be less than $3/p_0$ where p_0 stood for a predetermined population frequency which, for an accurate working for this formula, had to be equal or less than 2%. Our formula gave the required sample size that yielded the 95% confidence interval, $p<3/n$. Thus if the frequency of Behçet's syndrome (BS) is around 1/250 among the adult population in Turkey and we do a survey BS in the UK and do not come across a single patient among 750 individuals we can conclude that the prevalence of BS in UK is less than that in Turkey with 95% confidence.

It is also proposed that the frequency of the disease in the region where the disease is thought to have low prevalence can be estimated by a "neighbourhood sample", instead of the traditional random sample of the population. Assuming that we do not come across any cases, even in this setting of the worst case conditions, than we can be more comfortable in the upper boundary that our zero patient formula will define.

KEYWORDS: Zero – patient method; epidemiology; neighbourhood sample; confidence limits

INTRODUCTION

Reliable figures related to the frequency of Behçet's syndrome (BS) are few. In the only formal population survey conducted by us some years ago in Turkey, we had come with a 1/250 among the inhabitants in a town in Northern Turkey [1]. What is needed, on the other hand, is an estimate of the frequency of this condition in the areas, like Europe and North America, where the disease is apparently much less common. This is particularly important in trying to compare the frequency of BS among the indigenous people of these countries and that among the immigrants from areas with a high prevalence of BS, like Turkey and Japan. Such studies are obviously important to tease out the acquired from the genetic components in the pathogenesis of BS, about which relatively little is yet known.

It is proposed that the utilisation of our recently published "zero patient" method [2] of statistical analysis and the neighbourhood method of selecting the population to be studied will facilitate such studies.

THE ZERO PATIENT METHOD

To formally study the epidemiology of rare diseases is often difficult and costly in that large number of patients need to be studied. There is also the, not well-recognised, problem of not being able to the formal statistics in the, rather likely, event that no patients with the rare disease under scrutiny is identified among the several hundred or thousand individuals screened. Several colleagues versed in statistics and mathematics and myself recently proposed a method to address this problem [2]. The mean objective was to determine an upper boundary for "zero" observations among a population of "n" individuals.

Using the binomial distribution model, the upper limit of "n" was formulated to be less than $3/p_0$ where p_0 stood for a predetermined population frequency which, for an accurate working for this formula, had to be equal or less than 2%. Our formula gave the required sample size that yielded the 95% confidence interval $p<3/n$.

Let us look at a numerical example:

We mentioned that the frequency of Behçet's syndrome (BS) is around 1/250 among the adult population in Turkey [1]. Assuming we do a survey BS in the United Kingdom and do not come across a single patient among 750 ($3\times1/250$) we come across. With this observation we can safely conclude that the prevalence of BS in UK is less than that in Turkey with 95% confidence. Similarly, in 1998 Sezer at all screened 45000 children in Turkey and could not come across a single patient with BS [3]. This told us that the frequency of BS, among children in Turkey was less than 1/15000, with 95% confidence. This certainly is in line with the traditional view that BS is rare among children.

One final point that needs to be discussed about our formula is its power. This simply is the likelihood that we will find "zero" cases if we formally do the mentioned survey with our upper bound number of our frequency being defined as $3/p_0$. For an 80% power this frequency is around 13 times less than p_0. Let us assume that the frequency of BS in UK is less than $1/13\times250$. The power of our test tells that if we survey 100 random and different samples of individuals in UK, 80 out of 100 times we will not come across any patients with BS.

We believe that this 13-fold difference is rather comfortable, and thus the power of our formula quite acceptable in that the true prevalence of BS in UK, in all likelihood, is even less than $1/13\times250$.

Hasan Yazici

As mentioned above the main reason our formula was designed was to use it in comparative studies between a region of relatively high disease prevalence and that in a region where the frequency is very low.

It is proposed that the frequency of the disease in the region where the disease is thought to have low prevalence can be estimated by a "neighbourhood sample", instead of the traditional random sample of the population. This neighbourhood sample would be people among the immediate vicinity of the already identified cases. Such a sample would be biased toward finding more cases than what one would expect in a traditional random sample simply due to an augmented influence of environmental and/or genetic factors operative in the pathogenesis in a neighbourhood sample. However, assuming that we do not come across any cases, even in this setting of the worst case conditions, than we can be more comfortable in the upper boundary that our zero patient formula will define.

An operational example of this method would be to start with a case registry of BS patients in Northern European country where BS is known to be very rare. The next step would be to search for other cases of BS in the immediate, well-defined, vicinity of these cases. This "vicinity" could, for example, be the work place or the dwelling of the already identified cases. The relatives may or may not be included in this survey as we wish.

Another point to consider in this proposed method is the intuitively expected similarity of environmental agents or individual traits in disease causation in different geographic areas. This would make the comparisons in frequency arrived by our method, in probability, be valid in that one would reasonably expect more or less similar factors of disease causation in different regions.

CONCLUSION

It is suggested that utilisation of the "neighbourhood sample" with the "zero-patient method" will ease our way to make comparative studies on the frequency of rare diseases less costly and time consuming.

REFERENCES

1. Yurdakul, S, Günaydin, I, Tüzün Y. et al. *J. Rheumatol.* 15:820–2, 1988.
2. Yazici, H, Biyikli, M, van der Linden, S Schouten H.J.A. *Rheumatol.* 40:121–22, 2001.
3. Özen, S, Karaaslan, Y Özdemir O. et al. *J. Rheumatol.* 25:2445–9, 1998.

FEREYDOUN DAVATCHI, FARHAD SHAHRAM, CHEYDA CHAMS, HORMOZ CHAMS, ABDOL-HADI NADJI, AHMAD-REZA JAMSHIDI, MAHMOOD AKBARIAN AND FARHAD GHARIBDOOST

3. Non-Ocular Manifestations

ABSTRACT

Behçet's Disease (BD) is classified among vasculitides. There are actually two nation-wide surveys of BD; Iran (3153 patients) and Japan (3316 patients). There are 4 major case series in the world, Turkey (2147 patients), Korea (1155 patients), Morocco (673 patients), and England (419 patients). Other series are based on less than 200 patients.

Mucous Membrane Manifestations: *Oral aphthosis* was seen in 96.4% of patients in Iran, 98.2% in Japan, 100% in Turkey, 97.5% in Korea, 100% in Morocco, and 100% in England. *Genital aphthosis* is seen less frequently. It was detected in 64.8% in Iran, 73.2% in Japan, 88.2% in Turkey, 56.7% in Korea, 83.5% in Morocco, and 89% in England.

Skin Manifestations: They were seen in 71.8% of patients in Iran, 87.1% in Japan, 60.6% in Korea, and 86% in England. *Behçet's Pustulosis* or pseudo-folliculitis was seen in 63.7% of patients in Iran. *Skin aphthosis* is not frequent but it is the most characteristic lesion of BD. *Subcutaneous Lesions*: Erythema nodosum is seen in 22.6% of patients in Iran. They are seen more frequently in China and Korea, around 55% of patients.

Ocular Manifestations: they were seen in 56.2% of patients in Iran, in 69% in Japan, 28.9% in Turkey, 28.5% in Korea, 67% in Morocco, and 68% in England. Anterior uveitis was seen in 41.8% of patients in Iran, posterior uveitis in 44.9%, and retinal vasculitis in 30.9% of patients.

Joint Manifestations: They were seen in 36% of patients in Iran, 57% in Japan, 16% in Turkey, 24.2% in Korea, 56.9% in Morocco, and 93% in England. They have different forms: Arthralgia, monoarthritis, Oligo/poly arthritis, and Ankylosing spondylitis.

Neurological manifestations: were seen in 9.5% of patients in Iran, 11% in Japan, 2.2% in Turkey, 5.7% in Korea, 14% in Morocco, and 31% in England.

Gastrointestinal (GI) manifestations: Produced by aphthous ulcers of the intestinal tract, they were seen in 8.1% of patients in Iran, 15.5% in Japan, 2.8% in Turkey, 4% in Korea, and 7% in England.

Vascular involvement was seen in 8.4% of cases in Iran, 8.9% in Japan, and 16.8% in Turkey. Arterial involvement is rarely seen, In Iran it was 0.5% of patients. Deep vein thrombosis was seen in 6% of patients in Iran, 8.9% in Japan, 10.6% in Turkey, 19.2% in Morocco, and 22% in England. Superficial phlebitis was seen in 2.3% of patients in Iran. Large vein thrombosis was seen in 0.9% of patients in Iran

Orchitis, Epididymitis were seen in 5.8% of patients in Iran, and 6% in Japan. Cardio Pulmonary manifestations were rare.

Laboratory Findings: Erythrocyte Sedimentation rate was normal in 41.2% of cases in Iran. Urinary abnormalities are infrequent and transient (10.3% of cases in Iran). Proteinuria was seen in 2.2%, hematuria in 4.7%, leukocyturia in 5.5%, and cast in 0.3% of cases. Pathergy test was positive in 59.5% of patients in Iran, 44% in Japan, 57% in Turkey, 40% in Korea, 68% in Morocco, and 32% in England.

KEYWORDS: Behçet's Disease, Clinical Manifestations; Muco-cutaneous Manifestations, Aphthous Ulcers

INTRODUCTION

Behçet's Disease (BD) is classified among vasculitides, but its clinical picture is very distinctive and can be easily differentiated from the others. Originally BD was seen along the Silk Road, but due to immigrations it is now seen everywhere in the world. There are many reports on clinical manifestations of BD from different parts of the world. The majority are case series reports. There are actually two nationwide surveys of BD, one from Iran [1] and the other from Japan [2]. Although the two countries are far from each other, and their populations are racially different, the difference between their clinical pictures was not striking [3]. Each of these studies was done on a great number of patients, 3153 patients for Iran and 3316 patients for Japan. The comparison of case series with the nationwide surveys is difficult because of the difference in patients' selection. There are 4 major case series in the world, Turkey with 2147 patients [4], Korea with 1155 patients [5], Morocco with 673 patients [6], and England with 419 patients [7]. Other series are based on less than 200 patients [8–26]. Looking at reports from all over the world, it appears that the clinical picture varies from one to another. These differences have led some authors to stipulate that BD was a syndrome rather than a disease. However, difference in selection methods and clinical settings may explain the majority of them.

The clinical picture of BD is dominated by mucocutaneous and ophthalmological manifestations. The criteria used in different sets of diagnosis criteria are for the majority among those manifestations. We will give a clinical description of each manifestation, and give their prevalence in major studies. The figures will then be compared to other statistics from other parts of the world (Table 1). The data from Iran are the latest figures compiled from our database in August 2000. The figures are driven from 4313 patients.

Fereydoun Davatchi et al.

Table 1 Distribution of Behçet's Disease clinical symptoms in the world.

	No.	OA	GA	Skin	Oph	Joint	CNS	GI	Phl	Epid
Japan[2]	3316	98	73	87	69	57	11	16	9	6
Korea[5]	1155	98	57	61	29	24	5.7	4		
China[8]	98	100	89		21.4	30.6	9.2	36		
India[9]	58	90	78	64	43	71			10	
Saudi Arabia[10]	119	100	87	57	65	37	44	4	25	4
Iraq[11]	58	100	100	83	35	31	19	3.3	33	14
Jordan[12]	150	100	85	90	46		28	20	29	28
Lebanon[13]	100	95	78	53	63	65	14	10	9	2
Israel[14]	41	98	88	88	76	29	29		37	6
Egypt[15]	274	92	76	39	76	50	26	10		16
Algeria[16]	58						14	5	21	
Tunisia[17]	200	100	80		60	50	20			
Morocco[6]	673	100	84		67	57	14		19	
Iran	4313	96	65	72	56	36	3.3	8	6	6
Turkey[4]	2147	100	88		29	16	2.2	2.8	11	
Tadjikistan[18]	36	100	71	79	49	44	14		14	
Russia[19]	35	100	89	89	40	71	14	37	37	4
Greece[20]	90	100	77	74	71	56	20			11
Italy[21]	155	98	73	86	92	77	17	34	18	19
Portugal[22]	127	98	75		87	55				
Spain[55]	38	100	91	73	35	62	17	5	19	
Germany[23]	196	99	75	76	59	59	13	16		16
France[24]	73	97	62	74	55	94	28	18		1
England[7]	419	100	89	86	68	93	31	7	22	
USA[25]	164	98	80	66	70	42	21	8		2
Brazil[26]	81	100	71	65	51	64				7

No.: Number of cases. *OA:* Oral aphthosis. *GA:* Genital aphthosis.
Oph: Ophthalmologic Manifestations. *CNS:* Central nervous system involvement.
GI: Gastrointestinal manifestations. *Phl:* Phlebitis. *Epid:* Epididymitis.

MUCOUS MEMBRANE MANIFESTATIONS

Classically they are oral and genital aphthosis. The two of them are used in diagnosis criteria. However, other lesions can be seen which are ulcerations but not aphthosis.

Oral aphthosis is the most frequent and constant symptom of BD. It was seen in 96.4% of patients in Iran (Confidence Interval: 0.5) 98.2% in Japan (CI: 0.5), 100% in Turkey, 97.5% in Korea, 100% in Morocco, and 100% in England. Oral aphthosis is not specific to BD and can be seen in other diseases like AIDS, ulcerative colitis, Crohn disease, systemic lupus erythematosus, etc. The elementary lesion is a well-

defined and painful round or oval ulceration. It has a white yellowish necrotic base, surrounded by a red areola. The number of aphthous lesions varies from one attack to another. Sometimes it is isolated, but most of the time two or more lesions are seen together. The diameter of lesions varies from one attack to another, from 1 to 20 mm, with a tendency to decrease under the treatment. The lesions heal spontaneously in one or two weeks, without any treatment, but they have a high tendency for recurrence. The interval between recurrences also varies from one attack to another, from few days to several months, or even more. Classically, oral aphthosis is classified in major, minor, and herpetiform aphthosis. This classification is no more relevant, because there is no fundamental difference between them. If the size of aphthous lesions or their grouping has to be considered then the following forms can be described:
– Punctiform aphthous lesions: They are very small, like a pinhole. They are some-time difficult to see because of their small size. However, as they are painful and the patient will usually point at them, their detection becomes easier. Usually a few of them may be detected at the same time.
– The miliaria aphthosis are small and numerous aphthous lesions usually seen on the lips and cheeks. The differential diagnosis is the Fordyce spots, which are not painful and do not disappear like aphthous lesions.

Oral aphthous lesions may be localized everywhere on the oral mucosa with the following frequency order: lips, cheeks, tongue, gingiva, palate, tonsils, and pharynx. Different forms of oral aphthous lesions may be seen together at the same time. Giant aphthous lesions are rare in oral mucosa, but more frequent in genitalia.

Genital aphthosis is seen less frequently than oral aphthosis. It was detected in 64.8% in Iran (CI: 1.4), 73.2% in Japan, 88.2% in Turkey, 56.7% in Korea, 83.5% in Morocco, and 89% in England. The clinical picture is like oral aphthosis, except lesion are usually more large, heal more slowly, and recur less frequently. In females they are often larger than 10 mm, and deeper than oral aphthous lesions. They are localized on the vulva, vagina, and rarely cervix. The giant aphthous lesion of the vulva is frequent, cause dysfunction, and sometimes leaves indelible cicatrix. In males, genital aphthosis is more often seen on the scrotum. They may sometimes become giant lesions. Aphthous lesions may also be seen on the shaft of penis or on the meatus.

Other forms of mucous membrane manifestations include [27]:
– Anal aphthosis: This peculiar and rare form of aphthosis can be seen in both sexes. It has the same characteristic than the genital aphthosis. The lesion is external and close to the sphincter.
– Conjunctival aphthosis: This is also a rare lesion. Most of the time it is missed, because it is small and ephemera, while the internal eye lesions may also mask the symptoms.
– Ulceration and erosions: They are different from aphthous lesions as they have different clinical characteristics. Ulcerative lesions are sometimes isolated and the cause may be difficult to diagnose. More often, they are seen together with the common aphthosis. The ulceration can produce multiple and various shapes with-out a specific characteristic.
  – Fissural form.
  – Punctuated form.

- Slashed form.
- Open book, like superficial ulceration.
- Giant ulceration.

These lesions were seen rarely. Without histological proof, the superficial and confluent forms are difficult to differentiate from the early stage of pemphigus vulgaris. Before involving the skin, Pemphigus vulgaris can sometimes involve buccal mucosa for several months.

- Erythema: They usually surround aphthous lesions. They can also be isolated involving a large surface of the oral mucosa.
- Purpura and hemorrhagic lesions: Very rare, they may be isolated or be seen with other lesions. They are usually small and round, but they can also be widespread like a superficial hemorrhage.

SKIN MANIFESTATIONS

They were seen in 71.8% of patients in Iran (CI: 1.3), 87.1% in Japan, 60.6% in Korea, and 86% in England.

They have various forms. Pseudo-Folliculitis, Erythema Nodosum, and the Pathergy Phenomenon are the most classic.

Behçet's Pustulosis is a better nomenclature than Pseudo-Folliculitis. It is a vasculitis characterized by a dome shaped (non-acuminated) sterile pustule on a round erythemato-edematous base. The base may rarely become purpuric. Sometimes it can be seen around a hair follicle. Pustulosis is the most frequent cutaneous lesion of Behçet disease. It was seen in 63.7% of patients in Iran (CI: 1.4). It is seen mainly on the lower limbs and pubis, but it may be seen everywhere, even on the palmo-plantar skin. When it is situated on the face, trunk, and back, it can be mistaken with the papulo-pustular lesions of acne vulgaris by a non-experimented eye.

Small round erythemato-edematous lesion is characterized by a round and slightly painful weal on the skin, but without a pustule in its center like in Behçet's Pustulosis.

Skin hypersensitivity to traumatism (pathergy) is a frequent phenomenon. A skin trauma like needle prick will produce a papule or a pustule, surrounded by an erythematous reaction, at the site of the trauma. The pathergy test uses this phenomenon for diagnosis purpose. The skin is punctured with a 25 or 21-gauge needle, perpendicular or diagonally to the skin. The reaction is best seen 24 to 48 hours after the trauma. The degree of reaction which will classify the pathergy test as positive is not yet standardized; therefore the percentage of positive pathergy test differs from one report to another. However, it seems that in western countries, especially in England and in the USA, the frequency of positive pathergy test is lower than in Eastern countries. The pathergy phenomenon is not constant during the time and may appear or disappear during the course of the disease [28]. Pathergy phenomenon was frequently seen in Iran, 59.5% of patients (CI: 1.5). It was reported in 44% of patients in Japan, in 56% in Turkey, in 68% in Morocco, and in 32% in England.

Skin aphthosis is not frequent but it is the most characteristic lesion of BD. It is characterized by a yellowish narcotizing punched out painful ulceration. It is seen near the genital areas, on the inner side of the thigh, axilla, sub mammary space, interdigital spaces, buttock, peri-anal skin, and the trunk. Skin aphthosis usually leaves a round atrophic scar after healing.

Small nodules: They are indurated and painful dermis nodules. They are more frequently seen on the hands than lower limbs, but can also be seen on other parts of the body.

Behçet's cellulitis has been mistaken in the past with Sweet syndrome. It is a painful, large and round erythemato-edematous lesion. It is usually localized on the lower limbs, but sometimes on the upper limbs or on the face. It may sometimes mimic the clinical picture of Sweet syndrome's lesions. It must not be mistaken with the superficial thrombophlebitis of BD, or infectious cellulitis. The biopsy of Behçet's cellulitis showed always a vasculitis, and not a neutrophilic dermatitis [29] as in Sweet syndrome.

Pyoderma Gangrenosum like lesion: It is an exceptional lesion. It is a large super-ficial painful expanding ulceration, usually localized on the buttock and the lower limbs.

Subcutaneous Lesions: Erythema nodosum is the most important subcutaneous lesion of BD. It is rather frequent, and is a relapsing lesion. It is characterized by painful multiple subcutaneous nodules that have different sizes. They are preferential-ly located on the lower limbs. Often they have more erythema and edema around the lesions than the classic erythema nodosum. It is seen in 22.6% of patients in Iran (CI: 1.2). They are seen more frequently in China [8] and Korea [5], around 55% of patients. Other lesions are rare:

- Erythema Induratum like lesion is rare, 26 cases were seen in Iran. They are recurrent large subcutaneous, red mauvish, and indurated lesions resembling the erythema induratum of Bazin. The nodes become confluent, making a large indu-rated plaque. In some cases, there was an important widespread erythemato-ede-matous lesion. [29,30].
- Suppurative panniculitis is a very rare and special subcutaneous form consisting of recurrent episodes of fever with few nodes. These nodes become liquefied fol-lowed by the appearance of a fistula draining a sterile liquid. A localized atrophy with a round depressed region is left as a sequela. Five cases have been reported from Iran [30].

OCULAR MANIFESTATIONS

They are the major cause of morbidity in BD. They will be treated in detail in another chapter of the book. However, for the continuity of statistics, figures of eye involve-ment will be given here. Ophthalmological manifestations were seen in 56.2% of patients in Iran (CI: 1.5), in 69% in Japan, 28.9% in Turkey, 28.5% in Korea, 67% in Morocco, and 68% in England. The low figures from Turkey and Korea may be due to the clinical setting (Dermatology). Another report from Turkey gives the figure of 47.4% in a Rheumatology setting [31]. All parts of the eye may be involved, even conjunctiva and cornea. Anterior uveitis was seen in 41.8% of patients in Iran (1.5), while posterior uveitis was seen in 44.9% (CI: 1.5), and retinal vasculitis in 30.9% (CI: 1.4) of patients.

JOINT MANIFESTATIONS

They are not rare. They were seen in 36% of patients in Iran (CI: 1.4), in 57% in Japan, 16% in Turkey, 24.2% in Korea, 56.9% in Morocco, and 93% in England. Looking at another statistic from Turkey coming from a Rheumatology setting, the figure increases to 46.9% [31]. Joint manifestations usually follow the golden rule of attack and remission, although an attack may last several weeks or months. The main characteristic of joint manifestations is their favorable outcome. They may take any form. They can mimic from an acute and mobile arthritis like rheumatic fever to a chronic, fix, and additive arthritis like rheumatoid arthritis. A chronic polyarthritis leading to erosive joints is seldom seen.

Arthralgia, of inflammatory type is seen in 16.1% of patients in Iran (CI: 1.1), 9.8% in Israel [14], 62.4% in Morocco [32], 45% in Lebanon [13], 9.4% in Yorkshire [33], and 16% in Turkey [34]. Arthralgia is characterized by pain and morning stiffness while the physical examination does not detect any swelling. However, some joints may be tender.

Arthritis is usually monoarticular or oligoarticular. It affects mainly large joints with a predilection for the lower limb, much as the seronegative spondylarthropathies. Polyarticular arthritis, affecting small and large joint, mimicking rheumatoid arthritis is exceptional.

Monoarthritis was seen in 8% of patients in Iran (CI: 0.8), 20% in Russia [19], 3.4% in India [9], 18% in Lebanon, and 16.2% in Morocco [32]. Oligo/poly arthritis was seen in 17.6% of patients in Iran (CI: 1.1) and 51% in Russia. Oligoarthritis was seen in 34.5% in India, 23% in Lebanon, and in 11.8% in Morocco. Polyarthritis was seen in 32.8% in India, 11% in Lebanon, and in 17% in Morocco.

Ankylosing spondylitis (AS) is controversial. For some authors it is not seen in BD, while for others it is related to BD and is seen as secondary AS. In Iran AS was seen in 1.5% of patients (CI: 0.4), a number 15 times greater than in the general population. This data clearly shows that BD is one of the causes of secondary AS. In Egypt AS was seen in 5.6% of patients [35], in Iraq in 2% of patients [36], in Lebanon in 1%, in Morocco in 0.83% of patients.

In the study from Turkey [34], During a 4 year observation period (mean follow up time of 19 months) 26% of the patients had one or more attacks of arthritis, a total of 80 attacks for 47 patients. The knee joint was the most frequently involved, followed by the ankle, wrist and elbow. The mean duration of attacks was not calculated but 82% lasted for 2 months or less. The shortest attack was 3 days and the longest was 4 years. As for the outcome, the authors conclude that arthritis in BD is usually non-deforming.

NEUROLOGICAL MANIFESTATIONS

Neuro Behçet (NB) is an important manifestation of BD not because of its frequency, which is rare, but because of its severe morbidity and seldom mortality. The classic manifestation is a meningoencephalitis. However all forms of neurologic manifestations have been reported: from behavioral problems to organic confusional states, as well as seizures, headache, benign intracranial hypertension, diencephalic dysfunction, aphasia, pseudobulbar palsy, brainstem syndromes, cranial nerve palsies, hemiplegia, cerebellar syndromes, myelopathy, and mononeuritis multiplex may be seen.

NB was seen in 9.5% of patients in Iran (CI: 0.9), in 11% in Japan, in 2.2% in Turkey, in 5.7% in Korea, in 14% in Morocco, and in 31% in England (Table 1). If headache is set aside, the frequency of NB in Iran decreases to 3.1% (CI: 0.5).

A prospective study done in 1989 in Turkey on 323 patients followed for 1 year [37] showed an incidence of 14.2% (headache included). Patients with headache had no other neurological symptoms. Patients with neurological symptoms who could be classified as NB were only 5.3%.

Another prospective study was done in Iran in 1992 [38]. The study design was different from the Turkish study. In Iran study, 261 consecutive new patients referred to the Behçet's Clinic were evaluated. Among them 161 were classified as BD. The remaining 100 patients didn't have BD, although they were mimicking it. They were classified as control patients and were used in the study for comparison purpose. Headache was seen in 37% of BD patients and 43% of control patients. The headache was of tension type in 57%, vascular type in 28.5%, associated with attacks of mouth ulcers in 12%, and with attacks of uveo-retinitis in 1.5% of BD patients. The difference with the control group was not statistically significant. Minor neurological symptoms were seen in both groups with no significant difference. Major neurological symptoms were not seen in this group of patients who were at the beginning of their disease. Time and disease progression is important for neurological manifestations to appear. The Iran survey demonstrates that NB is extremely rare as the initial manifestation of BD. Usually it appears several months or years after its onset. Neurological manifestations are essentially due to the vasculitis of BD although other causes may be implicated [38]. Computed tomography scans were of little help for the diagnosis [37] and showed the same images in BD and control patients [38].

A retrospective study on 200 patients with NB [39] showed that 81% of patients had parenchymal involvement (hemispheric, brainstem, spinal cord), and 19% nonparenchymal involvement. The major manifestations in the first group were pyramidal signs, hemiparesis, behavioral changes, and sphincter disturbance. In the second group it was raised intracranial pressure due to dural sinus thrombosis.

GASTROINTESTINAL (GI) MANIFESTATIONS

They are not rare. Classically they are produced by aphthous ulcers of the intestinal tract, which may be situated on every part of it. GI manifestations were seen in 8.1% of patients in Iran (CI: 0.8), in 15.5% in Japan, in 2.8% in Turkey, in 4% in Korea, and in 7% in England (Table 1).

Fereydoun Davatchi et al.

The classical form of GI manifestations is the ulceration of the ileo-caecal region with symptoms varying from abdominal pain, diarrhea or constipation, proctorrhagia, to acute abdomen due to perforation of ulcers. However, ulcers are not localized only at the 2 extremities of the digestive tract. Ulcers can be seen all along the digestive tract with various clinical symptoms [40]. Dysphagia, retrosternal pain, and hematemesis are due to esophageal ulcers. Gastritis, peptic ulcers, abdominal pain, and diarrhea may be due to stomach and small intestine ulcers. Large intestine may also have ulcers, from the cecum and the ascending, transverse, and descending colon, to sigmoid, rectum and anus. The association of BD and ulcerative colitis has been reported.

Gastroduodenitis was seen in 3.1% (CI: 0.5) of patients in Iran, peptic ulcers in 1.6% (CI: 0.4), diarrhea in 2% (CI: 0.4), proctorrhagia in 0.8% (CI: 0.3), and abdominal pain mimicking surgical abdomen in 1.8% (CI: 0.4) of patients.

A prospective colonoscopic study of 46 consecutive BD and 27 Rheumatoid Arthritis (RA) patients [41] didn't demonstrate a significantly difference for the occurrence of lower intestinal involvement in them. However, aphthous ulcers were significantly more frequent in BD than in RA (26.1% versus 3.7%).

The main differential diagnosis of lower intestinal lesions is with Crohn's disease. Both have the same ulceration. However colonoscopic study of 94 BD patients with lower intestinal involvement and 67 Crohn's disease showed that ulcers in BD were usually round or oval, while in Crohn's disease they were mainly longitudinal. In case of a longitudinal ulcer, if it has a focal distribution it is mainly BD, otherwise (segmental or diffuse distribution) it is Crohn's disease [42].

VASCULAR INVOLVEMENT

They were seen in 8.4% of cases in Iran (CI: 0.8), in 8.9% in Japan, and in 16.8% in Turkey. They include arterial and venous involvement.

Arterial involvement includes thrombosis, aneurysms, and pulse weakness. They are rarely seen and all reports are unanimous on its rarity, except for Saudi Arabia with a rate of 18%. In Iran arterial involvement was seen in 20 patients (0.5% of patients, CI: 0.2). Arterial thrombosis was seen in 3 patients, aneurysm in 17 patients, and pulse weakness in 3 patients (lesions were cumulative, a patient could have more than one kind of lesion).

Deep vein thrombosis (DVT) is the main feature. It was seen in 6% of patients in Iran (CI: 0.7), in 8.9% in Japan, in 10.6% in Turkey, in 19.2% in Morocco, and in 22% in England. Symptoms and the outcome are the same as in phlebitis of other origin, but in BD phlebitis has more tendency to recur. Superficial phlebitis, although rare, is one of the characteristics of BD. It is segmental, appearing as a subcutaneous longitudinal swelling. It is transient, like the majority of BD symptoms, disappearing in a few days. Superficial phlebitis was seen in 2.3% of patients in Iran (CI: 0.4). Large vein thrombosis is seen less frequently than phlebitis. It involves mainly superior and inferior vena cava, but may also involve mesenteric, portal, hepatic, splenic, iliac, femoral, subclavian, and axillary veins. Clinical symptoms will vary depending on the site of thrombosis. Large vein thrombosis was seen in 0.9% of patients in the Iran (CI: 0.3).

If clinically vascular involvement is not very frequent in major reports, a systematic evaluation of 100 patients [43] with high resolution color duplex sonography in association with other techniques showed 79% vascular involvement (63% arterial involvement, 55% venous manifestations, and 39% both). Major arterial lesions were present in 33% and minor lesions in 48% of patients.

PULMONARY MANIFESTATIONS

These manifestations have different etiology; vasculitis, embolism, fibrosis, pleurisy, and infection. Although rare, pulmonary manifestations were the leading cause of death in BD, especially pulmonary vasculitis. Thirty-two cases (0.7%) were seen in Iran survey (CI: 0.2). Vasculitis was seen in 8 patients, fibrosis in 3 patients, embolism in 4 patients, pleurisy in 6 patients, infection in 12 patients, and other lesions in 7 patients.

CARDIAC MANIFESTATIONS

They are as rare as pulmonary manifestations. They were seen in only 20 cases in Iran (0.5%, CI: 02). Angina pectoris was seen in 4 cases, myocardial infarction in 4 cases, murmur in 7 cases, heart failure one case, and pericarditis in 5 cases. Multiple case reports can be found in the literature on cardiac manifestations describing every form of cardiac involvement.

A study on 30 cases of BD and 30 control patients [44] showed a higher incidence of mitral valve prolapse (50%) and proximal aorta dilatation (30%) in BD patients than in controls (6.6% and 0%). The difference was statistically significant. In another study 104 BD and 144 control patients were studied in a double blind case control study [45]. There was no statistically significant difference between cardiac symptoms and signs, ECG abnormalities, chest X-ray, and echocardiography abnormalities. Mitral valve prolapse was seen in 27% of BD patients and 17% of control patients (difference not significant).

ORCHITIS, EPIDIDYMITIS

They were seen in 5.8% of patients in Iran (CI: 0.7), and 6% in Japan. They were seen with much higher incidence (up to 28%) in some reports (Table 1). They have a low tendency for recurrence. The attack of epididymitis may be a painful or a painless swelling, lasting few days or weeks. The attack of orchitis is painful and affects both testicles.

Fereydoun Davatchi et al.

Urinary abnormalities are not frequent in BD. They are usually transient, but may become chronic in some cases. They were seen in 10.3% of cases in Iran (CI: 0.9). Proteinuria was seen in 2.2% (CI: 0.4), hematuria in 4.7% (CI: 0.6), leukocyturia in 5.5% (CI: 0.7), and cast in 0.3% (CI: 0.2) of cases. In 13 patients urinary abnormalities became chronic necessitating kidney biopsy. WHO type II was found in 3 cases, type III in 6 cases, and type IV in 4 cases.

One of the patients who had a WHO type III glomerulonephritis underwent a second kidney biopsy two years after the first one, due to aggravation of renal symptoms. Amyloidosis was discovered on the histology. Amyloidosis has been reported with much higher frequency from Turkey [46–47]. Since amyloidosis is exceptional in Japan and Iran, and considering that amyloidosis is very frequent as an inherited disease in Turkey, it may be concluded that the Turkish cases of BD and amyloidosis may be a fortuitous association of the two.

A case of renal transplant for an end stage WHO type IV glomerulonephritis was reported with a successful outcome at 28 months after the transplantation [48].

HEPATOSPLENOMEGALY

It was rarely seen; only in 22 patients in Iran (0.6%, CI: 0.2).

OVERLAP

An association with another disease may be seen. It may be difficult to find a relationship between the two entities. The association may be just fortuitous. An overlap or association was seen in 74 patients in Iran (1.7%, CI: 0.4).

LABORATORY FINDINGS

Erythrocyte Sedimentation rate (ESR) was normal in 41.2% of cases in Iran (CI: 1.5). ESR from 20 to 50 mm was seen in 34.3% (CI: 1.4), between 50 and 100 mm in 15.3% (CI: 1.1), and superior to 100 mm in 1.5% (CI: 0.4) of patients.

Pathergy test was positive in 59.5% of patients in Iran (CI: 1.5%), in 44% in Japan, in 57% in Turkey, in 40% in Korea, in 68% in Morocco, and in 32% in England. The rate of positive tests depends on the technique and the definition of the positive reaction. We use a set of 3 tests. 25-gauge needle with the intradermal injection of 1 drop serum saline, 25-gauge needle alone (no injection), and 21 gauge needle. The reaction is read 24 hours later. A papule formation at the site of the needle puncture with a surrounding erythema is required for positive reaction. The degree of reaction, which will classify the pathergy test as positive, is not standardized. Therefore the percentage of positive reaction differs from one report to another. Despite this, it seems that in western countries, especially in England and in the USA, the frequency

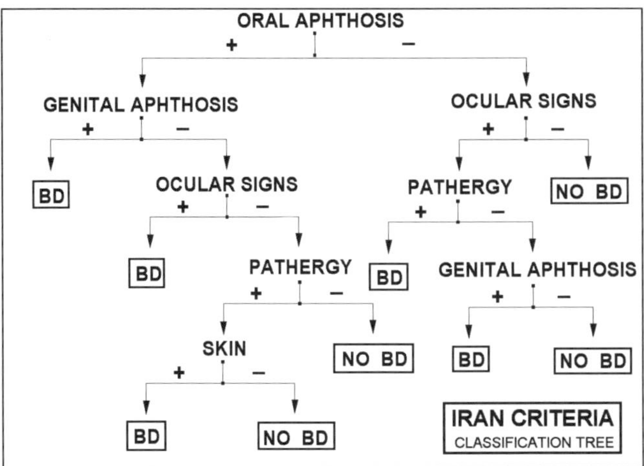

Figure 1 Classification Tree for diagnosis of Behçet's Disease.

of positive reaction is low. Beside the classical papulo-pustular reaction, in some patients a circular hemorrhagic reaction was noted. The hemorrhagic circle was centered by the needle prick, while the border of the circle was sharp [49]. In that study, the sensitivity of the pathergy test was 60.3%, the specificity was 86.7%, and the accuracy was 73.5%. The sensitivity of the circular hemorrhagic reaction was 12.3% and the specificity was 98.2% while the accuracy was 55.2%.

DISEASE CLASSIFICATION

The percentage of patients in Iran classified by different sets of diagnosis criteria were: Mason & Barnes criteria 69%, O'Duffy criteria 74%, International criteria 84%, Dilsen criteria 88%, Japan criteria 89%, Iran criteria (traditional format) 94%, and the Classification Tree 97%. Classification Tree (Fig. 1) has the best accuracy among other diagnosis criteria [50]. The accuracy of the International criteria was low. A recent study performed in China, in Iran, and in Korea on a standardized protocol confirmed the low sensitivity and the low accuracy of the International criteria versus Classification Tree [51]. The same was demonstrated in Russia [52] and USA [53].

DISCUSSION

The comparison between Japan and Iran surveys demonstrates some differences: In Japan survey there was a higher incidence for genital aphthosis (+8%), skin manifestations (+15%), ocular symptoms (+13%), joint manifestations (+21%), G.I. manifestations (+8%), and neurological manifestations (+8%). The difference may be due to differences in patients' selection, although racial differences cannot be ruled out. In Japan survey the patients selection was done by questionnaires sent to randomly

                                          Fereydoun Davatchi et al.

selected hospitals and the diagnosis was based on Japan criteria. This kind of selection may discard milder forms of the disease, increasing subsequently the percentage of all symptoms. For the Iran study all diagnosed patients all over Iran were included in the study and the diagnosis was not limited to a specific diagnosis criteria. The selection method in Iran permits the inclusion of mild forms of Behçet's Disease.

An analysis of BD in Turkey, Iran, Tunisia, Japan, and Korea led Dilsen [54] to the same conclusion (methodological, genetical, and environmental factors).

CONCLUSION

Behçet's Disease is a systemic disease with various manifestations. It progress by attacks and remissions. Lesions usually heal without sequela, except for eyes, brain, and vascular system. The main manifestations are muco-cutaneous. The major cause of morbidity is the ocular lesion, which leads to severe loss of vision or blindness.

REFERENCES

1. Davatchi, F, Shahram, F, Akbarian, M, Gharibdoost, F, Nadji, A, Chams, C, Chams, H, Jamshidi, AR, *APLAR Journal of Rheumatology,* 1: 2–5, 1997.
2. Nakae, K, Masaki, F, Hashimoto, T, Inaba, G, Moshizuki, M, Sakane, T in *Behçet's Disease,* Godeau, P, Wechsler, B (eds.), pp.145–151, Elsevier Science Publishers B.V., Amsterdam, 1993.
3. Davatchi, F, Shahram, F, Gharibdoost, F, Akbarian, M, Nadji, A, Chams, C, Chams, H, *Arthritis Rheum.* 38 (Supplement): S391, 1995.
4. Gurler, A, Boyvat, A, Tursen, U, *Yonsei Med. J.* 38: 423–427, 1997.
5. Bang, D, Yoon, KH, Chung, HG, Choi, EH, Lee, ES, Lee, S, *Yonsei Med. J.* 38: 428–436, 1997.
6. Benamour, S, Chaoui, L, Zeroual, B, Rafik, M, Bettal, S, El Kabli, H, Amraoui, A, *8th International Conference on Behçet's Disease,* Abstract P122, Reggio Emilia (Italy), 1998.
7. Seaman, G, and Pearce, RA in *Behçet's Disease,* Hamza, M (ed.), pp.196–199, Pub Adhoua, Tunisia, 1997.
8. Dong, Yi, Ming, Qiu Xiao, Zhang, Nai Zheng, Li, Cui Hai, and Wu, Qi Yan in *Behçet's Disease Basic and Clinical Aspects,* O'Duffy, JD, Kokmen, E (eds.), pp.55–99, Marcel Decker Inc, New York, 1991.
9. Pande, I, Uppal, SS, Kailash, S, Kumar, A, Malaviya, AN, *Br. J. Rheumatol,* 34: 825–830, 1995.
10. al-Dalaan, AN, al-Balaa, SR, el Ramahi, K, al-Kawi, Z, Bohlega, S, Bahabri, S, Janadi, MA, *J. Rheumatol,* 21: 658–61, 1994.
11. Sharquie, Kh, Al-Araji, A, Al-Rawi, Z, Al-Yaqubi, O, Hatem, A, *9th International Conference on Behçet's Disease,* Abstract L06, Seoul (Korea), 2000.
12. Madanat, W, Fayyad, F, Zureikat, H, Verity, D, Narr, J, Vaughan, R, Stanford, M, *8th International Conference on Behçet's Disease,* Abstract P142, Reggio Emilia (Italy), 1998.
13. Ghayad, E, Tohme, A, *J. Med. Libanais,* 43: 2–7, 1995.
14. Chajek, T, Fainaru, M, *Medicine,* 54:179–196, 1975.
15. Assaad-Khalil, SH, Kamel, FA, and Ismail, EA in *Behçet's Disease,* Hamza M (ed), pp. 173–176, Tunisia, Pub Adhoua, 1997.

16. Berrah, A, Remache, A, Ouadahi, N, Ayoub, S, Hakem, D, Boudjelida, H, Bensalah, D, Kessal, F, Zemmour, D, *9th International Conference on Behçet's Disease*, Abstract P006, Seoul (Korea), 2000.

17. Hamza, M, Ayed, K, Zribi, A in *Les Maladie Systémiques,* Kahn, MF, Peltier, AP, Meyer, O, Piette JC (eds), pp. 917–947, Flammarion Médecine Sciences, Paris, 1991.

18. Shukurova, SM *9th International Conference on Behçet's Disease.* Abstract P007, Seoul (Korea), 2000.

19. Alekberova, Z, Madanat, W, Prokaeva, T, Yermakova, N, Poljanskaja, I in *Behçet's Disease,* Godeau, P, Wechsler B (eds), pp. 171–174, Elsevier Science Publishers B.V., Amsterdam, 1993.

20. Kaklamani, VG, Markomichelakis, N, Vaiopoulos, G, Papazoglou, S, Kaklamanis, Ph. *9th International Conference on Behçet's Disease.* Abstract L05, Seoul (Korea), 2000.

21. Valesini, G, Pivetti Pezzi, P, Catarinelli, G, Accorinti, M, Priori, R in *Behçet's Disease Basic and Clinical Aspects,* O'Duffy, JD, Kokmen E (eds), pp. 279–289, Marcel Decker Inc, New York, 1991.

22. de Souza-Ramalho, P, d'Almeida, MF, Freitas, JP, Pinto, J in *Behçet's Disease Basic and Clinical Aspects,* O'Duffy, JD, Kokmen E (eds), pp 291–298, Marcel Decker Inc, New York, 1991.

23. Zouboulis, ChC, Kotter, I, Djawari, DJ:, Kirch, W, Kohl, PK, Ochsendorf, FR, Keitel, W, Stadler, R, Wollina, U, Proksch, E, Sohnchen, R, Weber, H, Gollnick, H, Holzle, E, Fritz, K, Licht, T, Orfanos CE, *Yonsei Med. J,* 38: 411–422, 1997.

24. Roux, H, Richard, P, Aarrighi, A, Bergaoui N, *Rev. Rheum,* 56: 383–388, 1989.

25. Calamia, KT, Mazlumzadeh, M, Balbanova, M, Bagheri, M, O'Duffy, JD, *9th International Conference on Behçet's Disease.* Abstract L03, Seoul (Korea), 2000.

26. Montenegro, V, Carlotto De Abreu, A, Schaimberg, C, Roberto Gonçalves C *8th International Conference on Behçet's Disease.* Reggio Emilia (Italy) 1998, Abstract P143.

27. Chams, C, Mansoori, P, Shahram, F, Akbarian, M, Gharibdoost, F, Davatchi F, in *Behçet's Disease,* Godeau, P, Wechsler B (eds), pp. 359–362, Elsevier Science Publishers B.V., Amsterdam, 1993

28. Chams-Davatchi, C, Davatchi, F, Shahram, F, Akbarian, M, Gharibdoost, F, Nadji A in *Behçet's Disease,* Hamza M (ed), pp. 356–358, Pub Adhoua, Tunisia, 1997.

29. Chams-Davatchi, C, Davatchi, F, Shahram, F, Nadji, A, Akbarian, M, Gharibdoost, F, Jamshidi AR, *Ann. Dermatol. Venereo.l,* 125 (3S): 153–154, 1998.

30. Chams, C, Davatchi, F *8th International Conference on Behçet's Disease.* Abstract L11, Reggio Emilia (Italy), 1998.

31. Dilsen, N, Konice, M, Aral, O, Ocal, L, Inanc, M, Gul, A, in *Behçet's Disease,* Godeau, P, Wechsler B (eds), pp. 165–169, Elsevier Science Publishers B.V., Amsterdam, 1993.

32. Benamour, S, Zeroual, B, Alaoui, FZ, *Rev. Rheum,* 65: 299–307, 1998.

33. Chamberlain MA *Ann. Rheum. Dis.* 36: 491–499, 1977.

34. Yurdakul, S, Yazici, H, Tuzun, Y, Pazarli, H, Yalcin, B, Altac, M, Ozyazgan, Y, Tuzuner, N, Muftuoglu, A, *Ann. Rheum. Dis.* 42: 505–515, 1983.

35. Abou-Seif, M, Assaad-Khalil, S, El-Siwy, F, and El-Sawy, M in *Behçet's Disease,* Godeau, P, Wechsler B (eds), pp. 285–289, Elsevier Science Publishers B.V., Amsterdam, 1993

36. Al-Rawi, ZS, Sharqui, KE, Al-Hadithi, FM, and Munir, JJ *Ann. Rheum. Dis.* 45: 987–90, 1986.

37. Serdaroglu, P, Yazici, H, Ozdemir, C, Yurdakul, S, Bahar, S, Aktin E *Arch Neurol,* 40: 265–269, 1989.

38. Sikaroodi, H, Soroosh, S, Shahram, F, Akbarian, F, and Davatchi, F in *Rheumatology APLAR 1992,* Nasution, AR, Darmawan, J, Isbagio, H (eds), pp. 107–109, Churchill Livingstone Japan KK, Tokyo, 1992.

     Fereydoun Davatchi et al.

39. Akman-Demir, G, Serdaroglu, P, Tasci B *Brain,* 122: 2171–2182, 1999.

40. Plotkin, GR in *Behçet's Disease: A contemporary synopsis,* Plotkin, GR, Calabro, JJ, and O'Duffy JD (eds), pp. 239–299, New York, Futura Publishing Co. Inc. Mount Kisco, New York; 1988.

41. Kang, YM, Kim, GW, Bae, HI, Kim, NS, and Jun JB *9th International Conference on Behçet's Disease.* Abstract L43, Seoul (Korea), 2000.

42. Lee, CR, Kim, WH, Cho, YS, Kang, JK, and Kim JK *9th International Conference on Behçet's Disease.* Abstract L45, Seoul (Korea), 2000.

43. Assaad-Khalil, SH, Rafla, SM, Yacout, YM, Fadel, AM, Abou Seif, M, and Hamawy RA *8th International Conference on Behçet's Disease,* Abstract P84, Reggio Emilia (Italy) 1998.

44. Morelli, S, Perrone, C, Ferrante, L, Sgreccia, A, Priori, R, Voci, P, Accorinti, M, Pivetti-Pezzi, P, and Valesini G *Cardiology,* 88: 513–517, 1997.

45. Shahram, F, Eslami, M, Shakoori, B, Haydari, M, Nadji, A, Akbarian, M, and Davatchi F *8th International Conference on Behçet's Disease.* Abstract P92, Reggio Emilia (Italy) 1998.

46. Dilsen, N, Konice, M, Aral, O, Erbengi, T, Uysal, V, Kocak, N, and Ozdogan E *Ann. Rheum. Dis,* 47: 157–163, 1988.

47. Yurdakul, S, Tuzuner, N, Yurdakul, I, Hamuryudan, V, and Yazici H *Arthritis Rheum.* 33: 1586–1589, 1990.

48. Apaydin, S, Hamuryudan, V, Sariyer, M, Erek, E, Ulku, U, and Yazici H *8th International Conference on Behçet's Disease,* Abstract P158, Reggio Emilia (Italy) 1998.

49. Mansoori, P, Chams, C, Davatchi, F, Shahram, F, and Akbarian, M in *Rheumatology APLAR 1992,* Nasution, AR, Darmawan, J, Isbagio H (eds), pp. 111–113, Churchill Livingstone Japan KK, Tokyo, 1992.

50. Davatchi, F, Shahram, F, Akbarianm M, et al. In *Behçet's Disease,* Godeau, P, Wechsler B (eds), pp. 245–248, Elsevier Science Publishers B.V., Amsterdam, 1993

51. *APLAR subcommittee for Behçet's Disease. APLAR Journal of Rheumatology, 1:237–240, 1998.*

52. Prokaeva, T, Alekberova, Z, Reshetnjak, T, Kuzin, A, Kirkunov, V, Rabinovich, I, and Ermakova N *8th International Conference on Behçet's Disease.* Abstract P7.

53. Calamia K T, Davatchi F *9th International Conference on Behçet's Disease.* Seoul (Korea) 2000, Abstract P13, Reggio Emilia (Italy) 1998.

54. Dilsen, N *8th International Conference on Behçet's Disease.* Abstract P159, Reggio Emilia (Italy) 1998.

55. Torras, H, Lecha, M, and Mascaro JM *Med. Cutan. Ibero Lat. Am.* 10: 103–112, 1982.

NICOLE STÜBIGER, MANFRED ZIERHUT AND INA KÖTTER

4. Ocular Manifestations in Behçet's Disease

ABSTRACT

Introduction: Behçet's disease (BD) is a multisystem vasculitis (affecting both arteries and veins) of unknown origin, which is most prevalent in Mediterranean countries and Japan.

Ocular manifestations: Ocular involvement, frequently termed ocular BD, occurs in 60–80% of patients on average 4 years after disease onset. The primary manifestation in 50% to 87% of the BD patients may be unilateral and occurs most often as an anterior uveitis, the classic finding is a hypopyon-iritis, but later on, in most of the cases bilateral panuveitis with a chronic relapsing course is present. The essential finding of the posterior pole changes in patients with ocular BD is an occlusive, necrotizing, retinal vasculitis in the posterior pole.

Prognosis of visual acuity/Treatment: Visual loss is mainly caused by the occlusive retinal vasculitis. Despite immunosuppressive therapy various studies have shown a bad prognosis for the visual outcome in patients with BD. This suggests the necessity for new therapeutic approaches in the therapy of BD. Interferon-α has been shown to be effective in BD patients with panuveitis and retinal vasculitis.

Conclusion: Several studies revealed, that Interferon-α may be superior to the standard immunosuppressive treatments, with a quick anti-inflammatory action and restoration of visual acuity.

KEYWORDS: Behçet's disease; ocular manifestations; anterior uveitis; posterior uveitis; retinal vasculitis

INTRODUCTION

Behçet's disease (BD) is a multisystem vasculitis (affecting both arteries and veins) of unknown origin, which is most prevalent in Mediterranean countries and Japan. Its main features are oral and genital aphthous ulcers, skin manifestations such as erythema nodosum, papulopustules or leukocytoclastic vasculitis, oligoarthritis, peripheral vascular manifestations such as thrombophlebitis, thrombosis, aneurisms, neurological and ocular manifestations. The disease is associated with HLA B51 in 50–70% of the patients [1].

OCULAR MANIFESTATIONS

Ocular involvement, frequently termed ocular BD, occurs in 60–80% of patients on average 4 years after disease onset [1–4]. It is the inital symptom in 10% to 20% of the patients [1,3,4]. Recurrences are common and the recurrent attacks of ocular inflammation lead to severe, permanent ocular damage unless effective treatment is instituted. Each attack damages the eye, therefore loss of sight occurs in affected BD patients (4). The reported frequency of ocular involvement in cases of BD is 83% to 95% in men and 67% to 75% in women (4). The disease is more severe in men, and bilateral disease occurs in 80% of patients.

The primary manifestation in 50% to 87% of the BD patients may be unilateral and occurs most often as an anterior uveitis, but later on, in two thirds of the cases bilateral panuveitis with a chronic relapsing course is present [1–5].

Nongranulomatous inflammation with necrotizing obliterative vasculitis may be found either in the anterior or the posterior segment, or, more commonly, in both.

Anterior uveitis may be the only ocular manifestation in BD patients. Anterior uveitis is an inflammation, which is limited to iris and to the vitreous. The synonym of anterior uveitis is *iridocyclitis* [6]. In the literature, the classic finding in BD patients, is an anterior uveitis described as occuring together with hypopyon (accumulation of lymphocytes in the anterior chamber) (Fig. 1) in 30% of cases [1,3,5]. Nowadays, iridocyclitis occurs mostly in isolation, which is probably due to earlier and more aggressive treatment, which has resulted in dampening inflammatory responses.

The inflammatory response in the anterior chamber in BD is nongranulomatous nature. The patients often complain of redness, periorbital pain, photophobia, and blurred vision. Slit-lamp biomicroscopy examination reveals conjunctival injection, ciliary flash in the perilimbal region, cells and flare in the anterior chamber, and fine keratic precipitates.

In eyes with severe iridocyclitis, in which hypopyon is not seen by direct slit-lamp examination, a small layering of leucocytes can be observed in the angle by gonioscopy. This is termed angle hypopyon.

The anterior uveitis may resolve spontaneously over 2 to 3 weeks even if therapy is not instituted. It is explosive in nature, appearing very rapidly. Some patients with BD may change form feeling perfect one moment to having severe inflammation 2 hours later. However, this anterior segment inflammation may not be accompanied by posterior segment involvement.

Structural changes of the anterior portion of the eye, including posterior synechiae, iris atrophy, and peripheral anterior synechiae, may develop during the course of repeated ocular inflammatory attacks. The presence of peripheral anterior synechiae or iris bombe' from pupillary seclusion may lead to secondary glaucoma. Neovascularisation of the iris can occur as a result of posterior segment involvement (4).

Uncommon anterior segment findings are conjunctivitis with or without subconjunctival hemorrhage, episcleritis or scleritis, keratitis, and rarely, extraocular muscle paralysis [1,2,6].

Changes of the posterior segment include white cell infiltration of the vitreous body, ranging from a moderate number of cells suspended on the vitreous fibrils to a dense plasmoid reaction with sheets of inflammatory cells, especially during the acute phase. An isolated vitreous inflammation is not characteristic of BD.

The essential finding of the posterior pole changes in patients with ocular BD is an *occlusive, necrotizing, retinal vasculitis* in the posterior pole (4). In most of the patients retinal vasculitis occurs mainly affecting the retinal veins, which is pathognomonic for BD as it is the only systemic vasculitis affecting small and medium sized arteries and also veins. Other typical findings are venous and capillary dilation with engorgement. Involvement of the retinal vessels in the form of acute periphlebitis or thrombangiitis obliterans may lead to massive retinal (Fig. 2) and vitreous hemorrhage (4). Patchy perivascular sheathing (Fig. 3) with inflammatory whitish yellow exsudates surrounding retinal hemorrhages (Fig. 4) may be seen. They usually accumulate in the deeper retinal layers during acute episodes, while the overlying retina shows turbidity and edema. Retinal edema is present in 10% to 20% of the cases, especially in the macula (4). Retinal atrophy frequently is present afte the retinal exsudates and hemorrhage resolve, offering stark testimony to the prior ischemia. Sheathing of the veins often precedes sheathing of the arteries.Choroidal vascular involvement occurs as well, and choroidal infarcts are probably more common than is generally appreciated (4).

Severe vasculitis may lead to ischemic retinal changes because of vascular occlusion. This vascular occlusion causes tissue hypoxia, which stimulates the growth of new vessels of the optic disc (Fig. 7) or elsewhere. These neovascularizations can rupture and bleed causing the vitreous cavity to fill with blood. Bleedings into the vitrous can lead to organization with membrane formation. These membranes may contract and pull the retina, causing retinal wholes with subsequent retinal detachment.

The optic nerve is affected in at last one fourth of BD patients (4). Hyperemia of the optic disc with blurring of the margins (papillitis) is the most frequently observed lesion of the optic nerve (Fig. 5). Papilledema is not frequent, but it may occur as a result of microvasculitis of the arterioles supplying the optic disc (4).

Repeated inflammatory bouts are the major concern, with the most vision-robbing pathology located in the posterior pole, with fibrotic, attenuated retinal arterioles, narrowed and occluded "silver-wired" vessels, a variable degree of chorioretinal scars, retinal pigment epithel alternations, and optic nerve atrophy (Fig. 6) being the consequenses of repeated inflammatory attacks (4).

COMPLICATIONS

Due to the inflammatory changes in the anterior segment, development of secondary cataract and secondary glaucoma are possible [1,2].

In the posterior segment obstruction of the retinal veins and arteries, due to retinal vasculitis, may lead to neovascular glaucoma, to optic and retinal atrophy (Fig. 6), degenerative macular changes, e.g. macular hole, retinal neovascularization (Fig. 7), retinal detachment, and finally to phtisis of the eye [2].

PROGNOSIS OF VISUAL ACUITY / TREATMENT

Visual loss is mainly caused by occlusive retinal vasculitis involving superficial capillaries of the retinal periphery, macula and the optic disc. To date, treatment of BD is based on steroids, colchicine, and immunosuppressive drugs (azathioprine (AZA) and cyclosporin A (CSA)) [1–8,11]. Despite immunosuppressive therapy various studies have shown a bad prognosis for the visual outcome in patients with BD: on average, after 5–10 years, visual acuity is ≤ 0.1 in 50% to 74% of patients [2–5]. In one French study, from Coucherau and Massin in 1992 [1], visual acuity was impaired to ≤ 0.1 in only 16% of patients after an observation period of 6 years. But these promising results were achieved with high doses of immunosuppressive drugs (e.g. CSA 10mg/ kg bw per day), which in the longterm could cause unacceptable side effects such as renal insuffiency and secondary neoplasia.

This suggests the necessity for new therapeutic approaches in the therapy of BD.

Interferon-α has been shown to be effective in BD patients with panuveitis and retinal vasculitis [9–12]. From 1994 to now our group has treated 50 patients with severe ocular involvement (panuveitis/posterior uveitis/retinal vasculitis) with IFN-α2a [13]. The mean observation period was 26 months. The mean posterior uveitis score (BenEzra et al. [13]) fell by 46% every week (p<0.001), visual acuity rose from 0.56 to 0.84 at week 24 (p<0.0001) (Figs. 7 and 8) (see chapter 19).

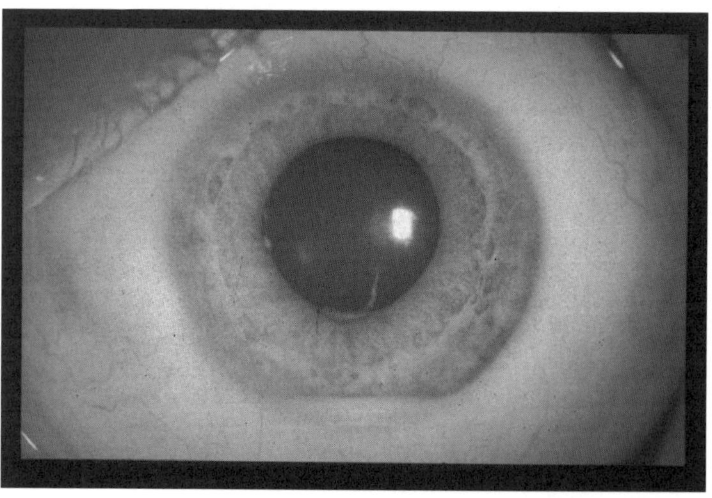

Figure 1 Acute Iridocyclitis with Hypopyon in a BD patient.

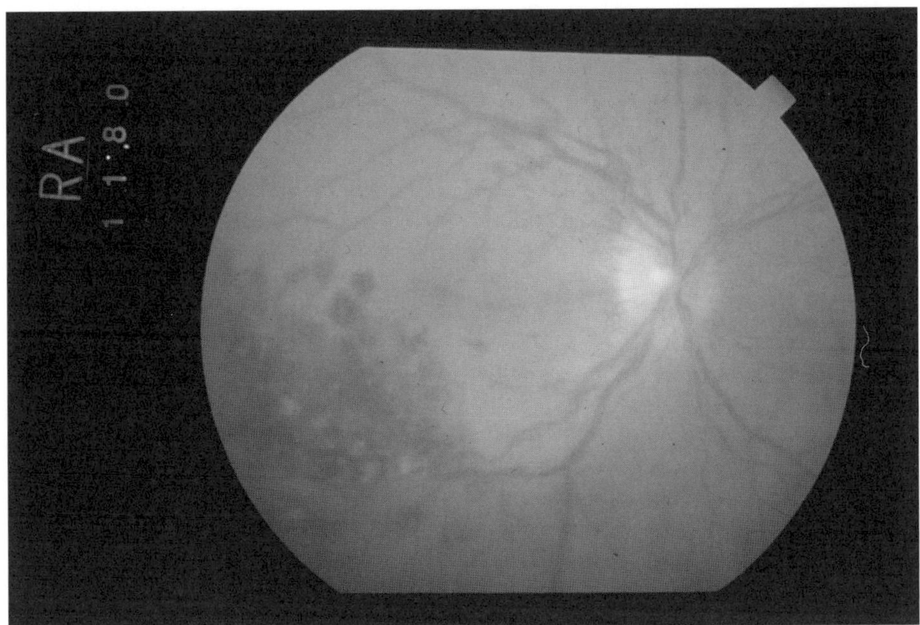

Figure 2 BD patient with a massive retinal hemorrhage due to a temporo-inferior venous branch occlusion.

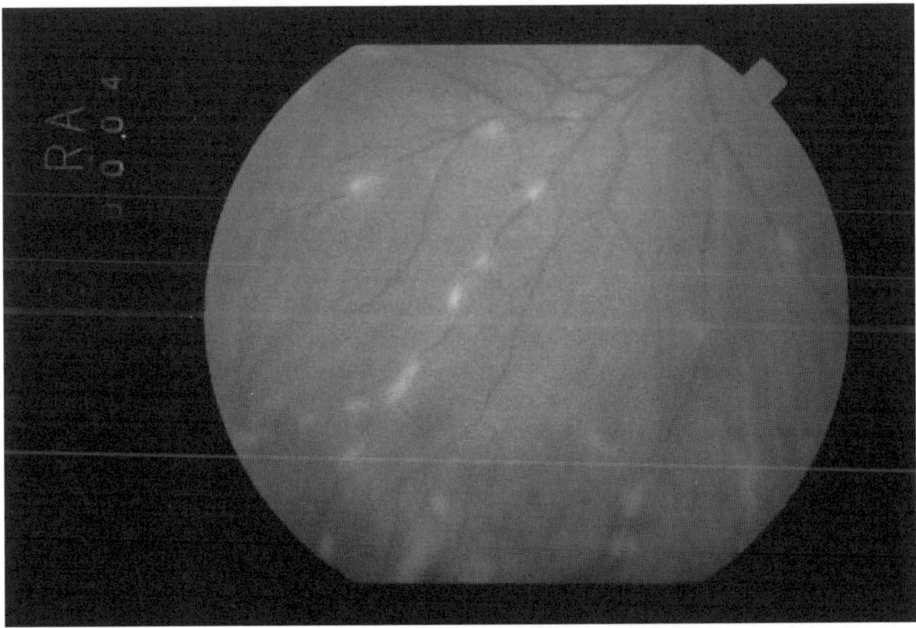

Figure 3 Yellowish-white perivascular sheathing and narrowing of the retinal veins in a BD patient.

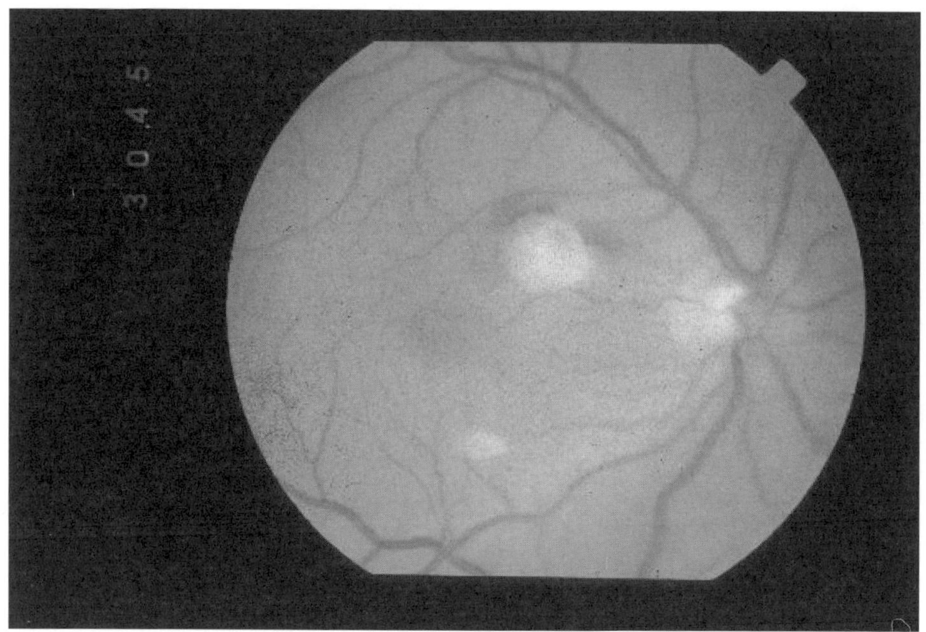

Figure 4 Inflammatory whitisch exsudates, the upper one is surrounding a retinal hemorrhage, on the posterior pole of a patient with BD.

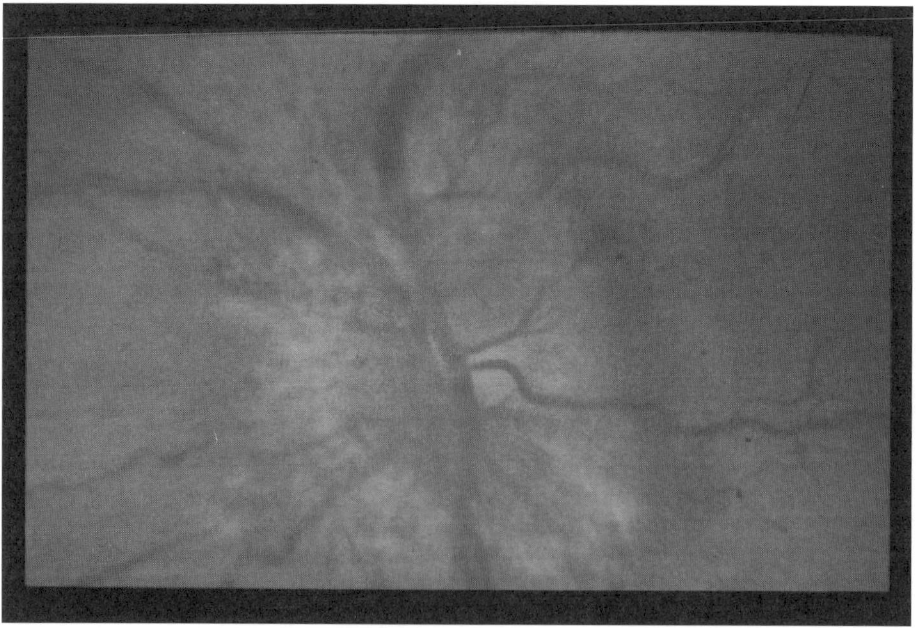

Figure 5 Acute Papillitis.

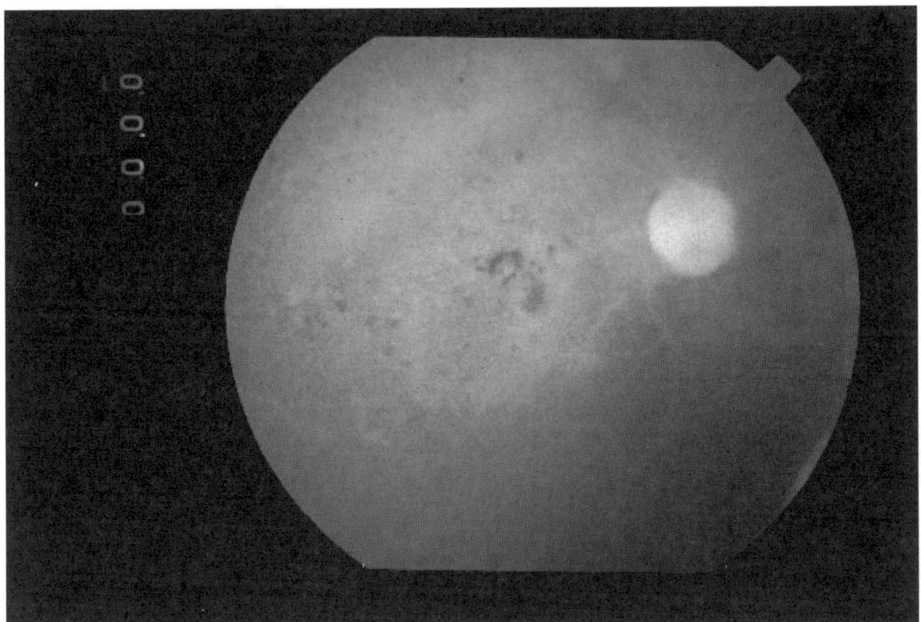

Figure 6 Fundus of a BD patient after multiple inflammatory attacks: narrowed and occluded "silver-wired" vessels, chorioretinal scars, retinal pigment epithel alternations, and optic nerve atrophy. Visual acuity: handmovement.

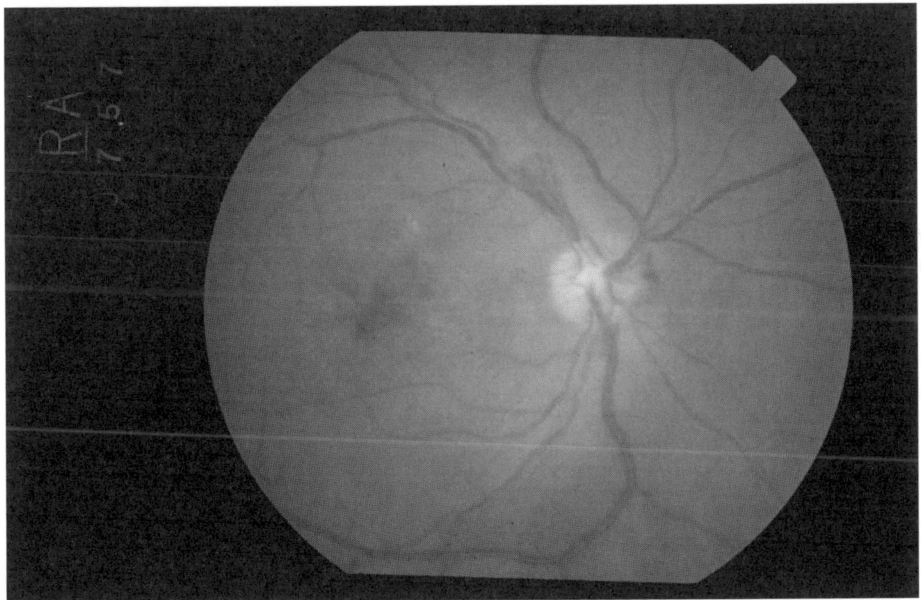

Figure 7 Neovascularizations of the optic disc, macular bleeding and edema, and dilated veins due to an acute inflammtory bout under therapy with Cyclosporin A. Visual acuity: 0.2.

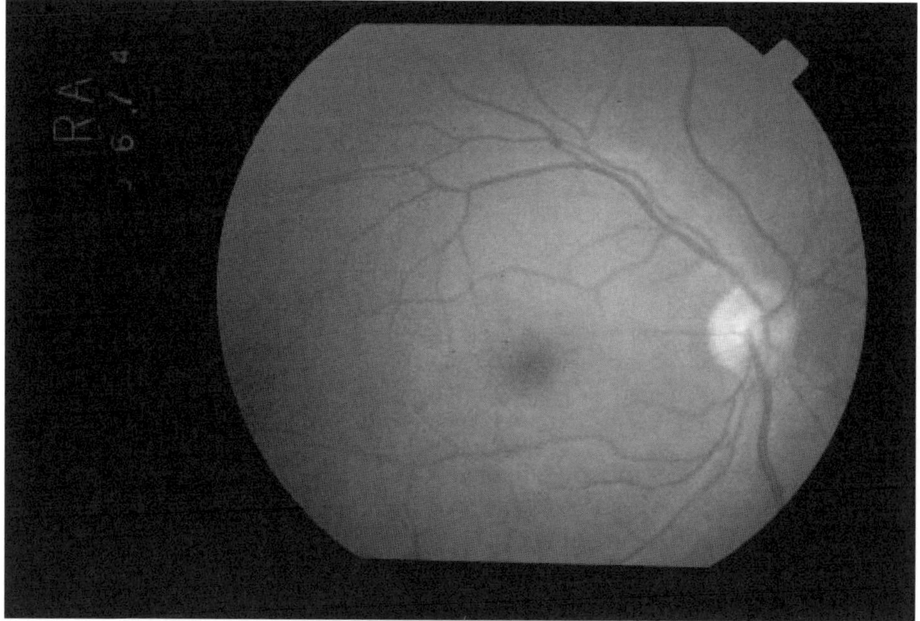

Figure 8 Fundus of the same patient as seen in Figure 7 half a year after beginning interferon treatment. The optic disc neovascularizations and the other inflammatory changes have completely disappeared. Visual acuity: 1.0.

CONCLUSION

In 60% – 80% of patients with BD, ocular involvement occurs on average 4 years after disease onset. The presenting symptom is anterior uveitis, but later on, in most cases, a bilateral panuveitis with a chronic relapsing course is present [1–5]. Visual loss is mainly caused by occlusive retinal vasculitis involving superficial capillaries of the retinal periphery, macula and the optic disc.

Despite immunosuppressive therapy, various studies have shown a bad prognosis for visual outcome in patients with BD [1–5]. Several studies revealed that IFN-α is effective in ocular BD [9–11,13] and it may be superior to the standard immunosuppressive treatments, with a quick anti-inflammatory action and restoration of visual acuity.

REFERENCES

1. Cochereau-Massin, I, Wechsler, B, Le Hoang, P, Huong LeThi, D, Girard, B, Rousselie, F, *J. Fr. Ophthalmol,* 15: 343–347, 1992.
2. Zierhut, M, Saal, JG, Pleyer, U, Kötter, I, Dürk, H, Fierlbeck, G, *German J. Ophthalmol,* 4: 246–251, 1995.
3. BenEzra, D, Cohen, E, *Br. J. Ophthalmol,* 70: 589–592, 1986.

Nicole Stuebiger et al.

4. Zafirakis, P, Foster, CS in *Diagnosis and Treatment of Uveitis*. Foster, CS, Vitale, AT Saunders Philadelphia 632–652, 2002.

5. Mishima, S, Masuda, K, Izawa, Y, Mochizuki, M, Nauba, K, *Trans. Am. Ophthalmol. Soc*, 77:225–279, 1979.

6. Zierhut, M Uveitis 1, *Differentialdiagnose*, Kohlhammer, Stuttgart, 2nd edition, 2001.

7. Kötter, I, Dürk, H, Saal, JG, Fierlbeck, G, Pleyer, U, Zierhut, M, *German J. Ophthalmol,* 5: 92–97, 1995.

8. BenEzra, D, Nussenblatt, RB, Timonen, P, *Optimal use of sandimmun in endogenous uveitis*, Springer Verlag Berlin, Heidelberg, New York, 1991.

9. Yazici, H, Özyazgan, Y in *Uveitis update: Medical Mangement of Behçet's syndrome*, BenEzra, D (ed.), pp.118–131, Karger, Basel, 1992.

10. Kötter, I, Stübiger, N, *Akt. Rheumatol*, 24: 51–57, 1999.

11. Kötter, I, Eckstein, AK, Stübiger, N, Zierhut, M, *Br. J. Ophthalmol,* 82: 488–494, 1998.

12. Kötter, I, Aepinius, C, Graepler, F, Gärtner, V, Eckstein, AK, Stübiger, N, Kaskas, A, Zierhut, M, Bültmann, B, Kandolf, R, Kanz, L, *Ann. Rheum. Dis*, 60: 83–86, 2001.

13. Kötter, I, Zierhut, M, Eckstein, AK, Vonthein, R, Ness, T, Günaydin, I, Grimbacher, B, Blaschke, S, Meyer-Riemann, W, Peter, HH, Stübiger, N, *Br. J. Ophthalmol.,* 87:423–431, 2003.

14. BenEzra, D, Forrester, JV, Nussenblatt, RB, Tabbara, K, Timonen, P, *Uveitis Scoring System*, Springer-Verlag, Berlin, 1991.

ELIZABETH D.E. KAISER, YILMAZ OZYAZGAN AND
NARSING A. RAO

5. Immunohistopathology of Behçet's Disease

ABSTRACT

Vasculitis is the immuno-histological hallmark of Behçet's disease and wide spread vasculitis characterizes the pathologic process. The ocular changes reflect a chronic, recurrent inflammatory process involving arterioles, venules and capillaries complicated by sequelae of inflammatory cell mediated tissue damage. The short-lived nature of the various lesions in Behçet's disease makes documentation of immuno-pathologic alterations most challenging.

KEYWORDS: Vasculitis; cell mediated immunity; retinal damage; hypopyon; visual loss

INTRODUCTION

Although Behçet's disease was originally described as a triad of recurrent oral and genital ulcerations along with hypopyon-iritis, the scope of the disease has widened over the years to encompass a spectrum of multiorgan involvement with variable manifestations. Hypotheses have been proposed as to its etiology, foremost of which is that an environmental insult triggers the disease in genetically predisposed individuals with the ensuing inflammatory disorder [1,2]. The role of HLA-B5 and its subtype HLA-B51 in the pathogenesis of Behçet's has been extensively investigated [3,4]. The high prevalence of HLA-B5 is most marked among patients living in countries located between latitudes 30° and 45°N [5], otherwise known as the Old Silk Route.

Microorganisms have been implicated as possible triggers of Behçet's disease due to its geographic distribution and varied manifestations in these areas [6,7]. Studies have mainly focused on herpes simplex virus (HSV-1) and Streptococcus (notably S. sanguis), but no definitive mechanism has been documented. Other organisms such as Hepatitis C virus and Parvovirus B 19 have also been studied but without establishing any causative correlation with the disease [3]. Results of microbial studies led to investigations of pervasive antigens, as the heat shock protein (HSP), which are able to initiate cross-reactive immune responses [8]. However, its pathogenetic role has yet to be resolved [3].

Organic compounds and trace minerals as chloride, copper and phosphorus have also been implicated in the development of the disease. Several studies have reported elevated levels of these compounds in the inflammatory cells, vascular endothelial cells, ocular tissues, and peripheral nerves of patients with the disease [9]. It has, however, not been determined if these elevations are a primary or secondary reaction to the ongoing inflammation.

IMMUNOPATHOLOGY

Vasculitis is the histopathologic hallmark of Behçet's disease. The characteristic feature of the active or acute inflammatory phase lesions is perivascular neutrophilic infiltration, along with scattered mononuclear cells [7,8,17]. Tissue injury is believed to be due to these neutrophils, which were observed to have enhanced chemotaxis, increased superoxide and lyzosomal production [8]. Perivascular lymphocytic and plasma cell infiltration are seen during remission [7].

Microbial antigens have been postulated to incite HSP with the consequent activation of macrophages [1] and stimulation of T-cells resulting in the production of interleukin-2 (IL-2), interferon-γ (IFN-γ), and tumor necrosis factor (TNF) [10]. The process likewise induces B cell proliferation. IL-2 is believed to augment IFN-γ production. IFN-γ regulates antigen presentation and activates the release of TNF-, IL-1, and IL-8. These factors, in turn, stimulate the expression of adhesion molecules on the vascular endothelial cells [3]. IL-8 being a chemoattractant [7] causes recruitment of neutrophils. Increased levels of IL-8 were found in patients with active disease, and the elevated level of this cytokine has been considered as a marker for disease activity [1].

Immunopathologic studies of both skin [7] and conjunctival [11] biopsies of patients with Behçet's disease revealed increased levels of CD4$^+$ T-cells and marked expression of HLA-DR$^+$, endothelial leukocyte adhesion molecule-1 (E-selectin), and intercellular adhesion molecule-1 (ICAM-1) with absence of the vascular cell adhesion molecule-1 (VCAM-1). E-selectin is an adhesion molecule involved in the preliminary entrapment of neutrophils from the circulation to the endothelium. ICAM-1, belonging to the immunoglobulin superfamily adhesins, brings about the firm leukocyte adhesion to the endothelium and controls leukocytic tissue migration [11].

$\gamma\delta$-T cells have been observed to be elevated in neuro-Behçet's patients and those with mucocutaneous lesions. However, their exact role is unclear. They may be responsible for cytokine production related to disease development [7]. Natural killer cells in peripheral blood of patients with active disease have been found to be increased, but with a decreased killing activity. This is thought to be related to the release into the circulation of immature forms of these cells [12].

Focal aggregates of B-lymphocytes, plasma cells, C3 and immunoglobulins (IgG and IgA) have been observed in ocular immunohistochemical studies [13, 14]. Circulating immune complexes have been implicated in the multisystem characteristic of the disease [15]; however, deposits of such complexes were occasionally observed in the renal lesions, episcleral, and some choroidal veins [14, 16].

ORAL ULCERS

Oral ulcers are considered the defining characteristic of this disease and are usually an initial symptom [6]. These painful ulcers occur in nearly every patient at some time during the clinical course. They can affect any part of the mouth but are found most commonly on the tongue, gingiva, labial and buccal mucosa. A typical lesion starts as a round, slightly raised erythematous area, which ulcerates in 1–2 days. It has a gray or yellow pseudomembranous surface with a necrotic white base bounded by a distinct erythematous halo. Healing occurs from 3–30 days, with or without scarring and recurrences are common.

Histologically, the area of the lesion exhibits eroded epidermis with dermal infiltration of neutrophils, lymphocytes and monocytes, particularly around the small vessels [16]. These vessels show intravascular aggregates of neutrophils with endothelial cell swelling, and fibrinoid necrosis surrounded by a mixed perivascular infiltrate of acute and chronic inflammatory cells [3].

GENITAL ULCERS

Genital ulcers are morphologically similar to oral ulcers, but are fewer, larger, deeper, more persistent and slower to heal. They are painful and recur less often than oral ulcers. These ulcers are commonly seen on the scrotum of males and the labia of females, but can occur in other genital parts. Histologically, these genital ulcers show features, which are virtually identical to those observed in oral ulcers.

CONJUNCTIVAL ULCERS

On rare occasions, patients with Behçet's may develop conjunctival ulcers. These morphologically show features of mixed inflammatory cell infiltration and prominent endothelial cells. Immunophenotypically the infiltrates constitute primarily $CD4^+$ T-cells. $CD3^+$, $CD67^+$ granulocytes, HLA-DR$^+$, and adhesion molecules E-selectin and ICAM-1 have also been documented [11].

SKIN LESIONS

Skin lesions can be grouped into two types, the papulopustular/acneiform/pseudo-follicultis lesions and erythema nodosum-like lesions. Recurrences are common. The most common skin lesions are the acneiform lesions. These lesions are usually seen in males, and are sterile. They can arise at any site but are commonly seen on the back, face, and neck along the hairline. They are morphologically similar to adolescent acne

[6], and can be seen in patients receiving corticosteroids [8]. These lesions are histologically viewed as leukocytoclastic vasculitis [16], which is characterized by polymorphonuclear leukocyte (PMNs) infiltration of small blood vessel walls, fibrinoid necrosis of the vessel walls, and fragmentation of the infiltrating leukocytes. Endothelial cell necrosis or hyperplasia [3] can also be observed. Pustular vasculitis and Sweet's-like vasculitis have been described.

Erythema nodosum-like lesions are painful, common in females, usually involving the legs, and resolve spontaneously leaving hyperpigmented areas. Histologically, focal small vessel vasculitis, perivascular lymphocytic and mononuclear infiltration, vascular wall fibrin deposition, endothelial cell swelling, dermal and subcutaneous inflammation can be seen [16]. These lesions, unlike the classic erythema nodosum, do not usually form histiocytic granulomas. Other typical findings include perivascular lymphocytic infiltration, phlebitis, lymphoid aggregates, and some fibrosis [3].

The pathergy test is used for assessing skin hyperreactivity, illustrating undue subacute inflammatory response to non-specific injury [17]. PMNs appear at the site of trauma in 6–12 hours, and at 24 hours there is significant infiltration of these cells as well as mononuclear and mast cells [16]. In addition, perivascular mononuclear cells are also observed in the deep dermis [3].

VASCULAR LESIONS

Widespread vasculitis characterizes the pathologic process of Behçet's disease. Involved vessels can be of any size in either arterial or venous systems, with frequent involvement of small vessels. It tends to occur in the early stages of the disease and is usually seen in men. Morbidity and mortality in Behçet's disease are attributed mainly to these lesions [1]. The most common venous lesion is recurrent superficial thrombophlebitis or deep vein thrombosis, which can give rise to thrombotic venous occlusion. Histologically, the obstructed veins may exhibit organized thrombi along with vessel wall lymphocytic infiltration and intimal fibrosis [16].

Arterial occlusion, though less frequent than venous, can involve any part of the arterial system. Thrombosis or stenosis may give rise to these obstructions. Histologically, the occluded vessel exhibits fibrous thickening of the media and intima [16]. Arterial aneurysm, involving the large arteries, is more common than occlusion, but they can coexist [16,17]. These changes are believed to be due to vasculitis, but may also result from trauma as a consequence of an invasive procedure. Prognosis is poor mainly because of the risk of rupture. Histologic examination reveals thickening of the intima, internal elastic lamina disruption, splitting and loss of the media elastic fibers, loss of the media muscle fibers and fibrosis of the adventitia. Proliferation of the vasa vasorum, along with lymphocytic, plasma cell, and PMNs infiltration are also noted [16,18].

CARDIAC LESIONS

Cardiac manifestations can be due to myocardial, pericardial, or endocardial involvement. Myocardial involvement is manifested histologically as degeneration of the myocardial fiber with mononuclear cell infiltration. Pericardial involvement is often seen during acute exacerbations. Histologic examination reveals granulation tissue displaying a mixed PMNs and mononuclear cell infiltration [16].

Endocardial involvement may vary from small vegetations on the valvular margins, to scarred perforated leaflets. Histologic manifestations depend on the disease stage. Vascularization, fibrin deposition, myxoid degeneration, and intense neutrophilic, lymphocytic, and macrophagic infiltration can be seen during the acute stage. Later, the infiltrate is mainly mononuclear with scanty neutrophils. Nonspecific valvular fibrosis can occur in more chronic cases [16]. Coronary arteritis, coronary artery aneurysms, and myocardial fibrosis have occasionally been observed [3].

PULMONARY LESIONS

Patients with pulmonary vasculitis typically present with hemoptysis. The vasculitis may be transmural mainly involving the large muscular arteries, mostly with a lymphocytic infiltrate [16]. The vasculitis can result in thrombosis, elastic lamina destruction, arterio-bronchial fistula, and aneurysm. [3].

GASTRO-INTESTINAL LESIONS

Gastrointestinal lesions are manifested primarily by ulceration at any point along the tract. PMNs, mononuclear, and lymphoplasmocytic infiltration, damage of the surface epithelium, and loss of goblet cells and crypts have been documented [3]. Esophageal ulcers reveal eroded mucosa, mixed inflammatory infiltrate in the submucosa, and granulation tissue at the ulcer base. Gastric ulcers show chronic inflammatory infiltrate of the lamina propria. Perforated ulcers may exhibit necrosis, hemorrhage, and perivascular mixed inflammatory infiltrate in the muscularis [16]. The ileo-cecal region is the typical site for the occurrence of gastrointestinal ulcers. Histologically, these and other intestinal ulcers show transmural inflammation made up of lymphocytes and destroyed submucosal connective tissue. A mixed inflammatory cell infiltrate is seen at the ulcer base [16].

NEUROLOGICAL LESIONS

Neurological involvement, known as Neuro-Behçet's, is generally associated with mortality in this disease [2]. It can involve any part of the nervous system and follows a variable course characterized by remissions and exacerbations. The main manifestations involve the brainstem and the pyramidal tract. Motor symptoms are more common than sensory. Seizures and headaches are also seen. The observed changes point to a non-specific inflammatory and degenerative disease, with neither selective nerve cell degeneration nor primary vascular changes [18].

The initial lesion is believed to be focal leukocytic infiltration, associated with perivasculitis and fibrinoid necrosis. Chronic lesions may exhibit perivascular and meningeal lymphocytic, plasma cell and macrophage infiltration. Perivascular fibrosis, parenchymal foamy cell infiltration, axonal degeneration and demyelination as a result of nerve fiber and myelin sheath destruction have been observed [16].

MUSCULOSKELETAL LESIONS

Muscle involvement in Behçet's disease has been classified into three types. The first type of muscle pathology exhibits muscle fiber degeneration, necrosis, and perivascular mononuclear and PMNs infiltration. The second type is neurogenic muscular atrophy wherein the muscle fibers are small, angulated and atrophic, associated with perivascular mononuclear cell infiltration. The third type shows normal histochemical profiles but with abnormal electron microscopy findings such as capillary basement membrane thickening, decrease in the lumen caliber, myofilament disorganization, and myofibrillary loss [16].

Skeletal involvement is typically self-limiting, non-deforming, monoarticular or oligoarticular disease predominantly affecting the knees. Histologically, the synovial superficial cell layer may be destroyed and replaced by inflammatory granulation tissue made up of lymphocytes, macrophages, PMNs, and fibroblasts [16]. Dilated venules and fibrin thrombi may be observed.

RENAL LESIONS

Different types of glomerulonephritis have been described including focal proliferative and necrotizing glomerulonephritis with patchy acute tubular necrosis, diffuse proliferative glomerulonephritis with epithelial cell crescent formation, rapidly progressive glomerulonephritis, and focal necrotizing glomerulonephritis.

Immunofluorescent studies reveal deposition of IgG, IgA, IgM, fibrinogen, and C3. Amyloid deposit in the glomerular basal lamina, causing nephrotic syndrome, has also been reported [16].

OCULAR CHANGES

Ocular involvement is regarded as the principal cause of serious morbidity in Behçet's disease [2]. It presents with various symptoms ranging from decrease in vision, floaters, pain, tearing, and photophobia to generalized eye redness. [8]. Onset is rapid; episodes are recurrent and explosive [6,17], lasting between 1–4 weeks, and usually resolving spontaneously. These repeated attacks, however, can lead to irreversible structural alterations, which can result in visual loss [8]. Visual loss occurs in 25% [6] of patients, approximately 5 years from onset of the ocular inflammation. Ocular involvement is the initial manifestation in 10–20% [3,6] of patients, and typically presents within the first 2–3 years from the onset of the disease [2,6]. It is more severe in men and is bilateral in 80% of patients [3].

The uvea and the retina are the usual sites of ocular involvement. Anterior segment lesions manifest as granulomatous or nongranulomatous iridocyclitis (Fig.1) with or without hypopyon [3]. Other anterior segment lesions include conjunctivitis, conjunctival ulceration, subconjunctival hemorrhage, keratitis, corneal ulceration, episcleritis, scleritis, and eyelid lesions. Retinal damage is characterized by vasculitis, vessel occlusion with accompanying hemorrhage, exudative lesions, edema, and neovascularization of the retina [6]. Vitreous inflammation and cystoid macular edema are also noted. Occlusive vasculitis can lead to infarction, necrosis, and atrophy of the retina, central or branch retinal vein occlusion, optic nerve atrophy and eventual phthisis bulbi may occur [2,19].

Ocular histopathologic findings are diverse. The most consistent finding is the marked intra-ocular vasculitis or specifically, the occlusive necrotizing nongranulomatous vasculitis and perivasculitis [2], most prominent in the early stage of the disease. The vasculitis has an obliterative and hemorrhagic pattern with necrotic changes, particularly in the retina [2]. Perivascular and diffuse neutrophilic infiltration, particularly in the uvea and retina, are seen during the acute inflammatory phase. The retinal vessels have swollen endothelial cells and thickened basement membranes. The vessels may show thrombus formation and eventual obliteration [20].

Inflammation, hemorrhage and cellular infiltration (Fig. 2) in all layers of the retina [16] after recurrent bouts of acute inflammatory attacks have been documented. Focal inflammation and perivasculitis in the retina cause areas of necrosis, which can ultimately lead to total retinal necrosis [14]. Perivascular lymphocytic and plasma cell infiltration in the uvea and retina occur during remission [3]. In the late stage, fibrosis ensues resulting in cyclitic membrane formation, and thickening of the choroid (Fig. 3) [20]. Optic nerve atrophy can result from perivascular lymphocytic infiltration in the optic nerve with axonal degeneration and replacement by fibrous astrocytes [16].

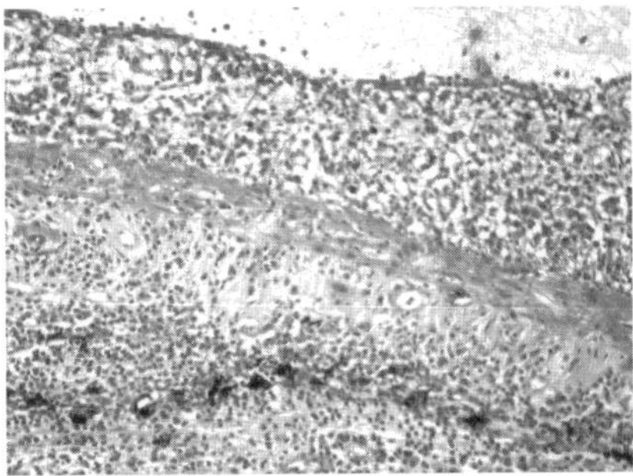

Figure 1 Markedly thickened iris from non-granulomatous chronic inflammatory cell infiltration.

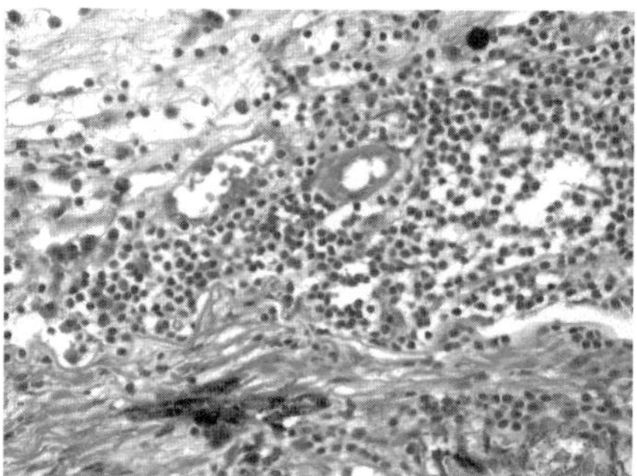

Figure 2 Gliotic retina with infiltration of chronic inflammatory cells.

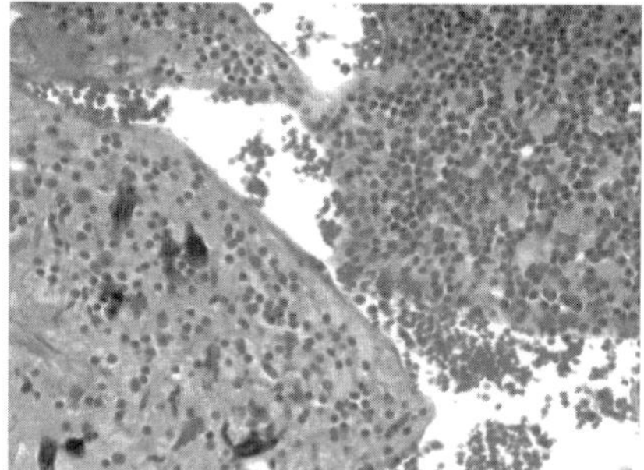

Figure 3 Thickened edematous choroid with inflammatory cell infiltration.

CONCLUSION

The immunohistologic and other histopathologic features reviewed herein describe the immunopathologic alterations observed mostly during the chronic phase of Behçet's disease. The ocular changes reflect a chronic, recurrent process complicated by various sequelae of inflammatory cell mediated tissue damage. Though vasculitis is regarded as the histopathologic hallmark of the disease, significant variations with absence of typical vasculitis may also exist. The short-lived nature of the various lesions in Behçet's disease makes documentation of immunopathologic alterations most challenging.

ACKNOWLEDGEMENTS

We wish to thank Ken Kaiser, Geeta Pararajasegaram, and Dr. Robert See for technical and photographic assistance.

Elizabeth D.E. Kaiser et al.

REFERENCES

1. Schirmer, M., Calamia, K.T., and Direskeneli, H., *J. Rheumatol.* 28(3): 636–639, 2001.
2. Bhisitkul, R.B. and Foster, C.S., *Int. Ophthalmol. Clin.* 36(1): 127–134, 1996.
3. Kaklamani, V.G., Vaiopoulos, G., and Kaklamanis, P.G., *Semin. Arthritis. Rheumatism.* 27(4): 197–217, 1998.
4. Yazici, H., Yurdakul, A., and Hamuryudan, V., *Curr. Opin. Rheumatol.* 11: 53–57, 1999.
5. Nussenblatt, R.B. and Palestine, A.G., *Uveitis Fundamentals and Clinical Practice*, p.213. Year Book Medical Publishers, Inc. Chicago, 1989.
6. Kontogiannis, V. and Powell, R. J., *Postgrad. Med. J.* 76: 629–637, 2000.
7. Hegab, S. and Al-Mutawa, S., *Clin. Immunol.* 96 (3): 174–186, 2000.
8. Sakane, T., Takeno, M., Suzuki, N., and Inaba, G., *N. Engl. J. Med.* 341 (17): 1284–1291, 1999.
9. Plotkin, G.R. *Pathogenesis: Miscellaneous Factors* in *Behçet's Disease: A Contemporary Synopsis*, Plotkin, G.R., Calabro, J.J., and O'Duffy, J.D. (eds), pp 89–98, Futura Publishing Company, Inc., New York, 1988.
10. Sohn, S., Lee, E., Kwon, H.J., Lee, S.I., Bang, D., and Lee S. *J. Infect. Dis.* 183: 1180–1186, 2001.
11. Tutkun, I.T., Urgancioglu, M., and Foster, C.S., *Ophthalmology,* 102(11): 1660–1668, 1995.
12. Powell, R.J. and Dunstan, S. *Postgrad. Med. J.* 67(788): 503–505, 1991.
13. George, R.K., Chan, C.C., Whitcup, S.M., and Nussenblatt, R.B., *Surv. Ophthalmol.* 42(2): 157–162, 1997.
14. Mullaney, J. and Collum, L.M.T., *Int. Ophthalmol.* 7: 183–191, 1985.
15. Haim, S., *Int. J. Dermatol.* 22:101–102,1983.
16. Lakhanpal, S., O'Duffy, J.D., and Lie, J.T., in: *Behçet's Disease: A Contemporary Synopsis*, Plotkin, G.R., Calabro, J.J., and O'Duffy, J.D. (eds), pp. 101–142, Futura Publishing Company, Inc., New York, 1988.
17. Pickering, M.C. and Haskard, D.O., *J. Royal Coll. Phys. London* 34 (2): 169–177, 2000.
18. Fukuda, Y., Uekusa, T., Watanabe, I., and Hayashi H., in: *Recent Advances in Behçet's Disease,* Lehner, T. and Barnes, C.G. (eds.), pp. 105–115, Royal Society of Medicine Services, London, 1986.
19. Lakhanpal, S., Tani, K., Lie, J.T., Katoh, K., Ishigatsubo, Y., and Ohokubo, T. *Hum. Pathol.* 16(8): 790–795,1985.
20. Kurumety, U., Okada, A., Usui, M., and Rao, N., *Behçet's Syndrome,* in *Ophthalmology,* Yanoff, M. and Duker, J. S. (eds.), pp. 10.18.1–10.18.4, Mosby International Ltd. London, 1999.

Immunohistopathology of Behçet's Disease

TOMOMI NISHIDA AND SHIGEAKI OHNO

6. T Cells in Behçet's Disease

ABSTRACT

The etiology of Behçet's disease is still unknown and it shows a lot of systemic symptoms. T cells are the most considered as a mediator in the pathogenesis of Behçet's disease. Especially, CD8+ γδ+T cells may play an important role and regulatory T cells have a possibility in the pathogenesis.

KEYWORDS: Gamma/delta T cells; CD8+ gamma/delta T cells; *Streptococcus Sanguis* (KTH-1), regulatory T cells

INTRODUCTION

Behçet's disease is a recurrent multisystemic inflammatory disease with symptoms of oral aphthae, ocular lesions, arthritis, and digestive tract ulcers. The etiology of Behçet's disease is unknown; however, the immunopathogenesis of Behçet's disease is considered to be mediated by T cells. The reports about T cells in Behçet's disease suggest that there are specific subpopulations of T cells based on whether their T cell antigen receptor is either an αβ or γδ heterodimer are involved in the pathogenesis of Behçet's disease. Here, we characterize some of the αβ+ and γδ+ T cells in Behçet's disease. In addition, we also suggest the possibility of generating regulatory T cells to suppress the pathology of Behçet's disease.

BACKGROUND

Normally, T cells recognize foreign antigens that are processed into short peptides and presented in cleft of major histocompatibility complex (MHC) molecules on the surface of autologous antigen presenting cells. This T cell recognition of presented antigen is mediated through the specific binding of the T cell receptor (TCR) to the presented antigen. The specificity of antigen binding lies in the variable and joining regions of the

TCR. By characterizing these TCR regions in human diseases with unknown etiology it may be possible to provide clues regarding the triggering stimulus.

Dr. Esin's group found in patients with Behçet's disease an expansion of peripheral blood CD4+ T cells expressing a specific beta chain TCR variable region (TCR Vβ) [1]. This was especially seen in patients with active disease. In addition, a particular beta-chain TCR joining region (TCR Jβ) was also expressed by the T cells. The expansion of these particular TCR Vβ-Jβ T cells correlated with disease activity. This has suggested the involvement of antigen specific T lymphocytes in the pathogenesis of Behçet's disease. Dr. Direskeneli's group found that the oligoclonal expansion of TCR Vβ-Jβ T cells in patients with Behçet's disease is in both CD4+ and CD8+ T cells populations [2]. They suggested that there is an antigen-driven oligoclonal expansion of T cells in Behçet's disease. Such findings open the possibility of applying immunoselective therapy for Behçet's disease.

αβ+ T CELLS

Activated CD4+ T lymphocytes can be considered to differentiate into 2 functional subsets, T helper type 1 (Th1) and type 2 (Th2) cells. The two T cell types have different cytokine production patterns and effector functions. Th1 cells produce interferon-γ (IFN-γ), interleukin-2 (IL-2), and tumor necrosis factor β (TNF-β). Th2 cells produce IL-4, IL-5, IL-10 and IL-13. Th1 cells mediate cellular immunity, and Th2 cells mediate humoral and allergic immunity. The balance of Th1 and Th2 cells responding to an autoantigen is known to be important in the induction and regulation of autoimmune disease. Th1 cells contribute to the pathogenesis of many autoimmune diseases, which can be suppressed by the activity of Th2 cells.

In Behçet's disease, there are several reports demonstrating abnormalities in humoral and cellular immune activity. There are high serum levels of IL-2, IFN-γ, and proinflammatory cytokines such as IL-1β, IL-6, TNF-α, and IL-8, in patients with active Behçet's disease. These results point to a polarized Th1 immune response. Dr. Frassanito's group has described elevated IL-12 in parallel with the increased percentage of IL-2 and IFN-γ producing T cells [3]. Their findings can be related to the prolonged inflammation seen in patients with Behçet's disease. Other reports have also shown Th1 cytokine levels are higher in patients with Behçet's disease [4]. Therefore, it is possible it is the proinflammatory cytokines produced by antigen-activated Th1 cells are responsible for the induction and pathogenesis of Behçet's disease.

γδ+ T CELLS

Besides αβ+ T cells, there are also T cells whose TCR consists of γδ dimers. This population of γδ+ T cells is a minor subset of T cells in humans. Although their function is unclear, γδ+ T cells are considered to be important players in innate host defense mechanisms and in autoimmune diseases.

                    Tomomi Nishida and Shigeaki Ohno

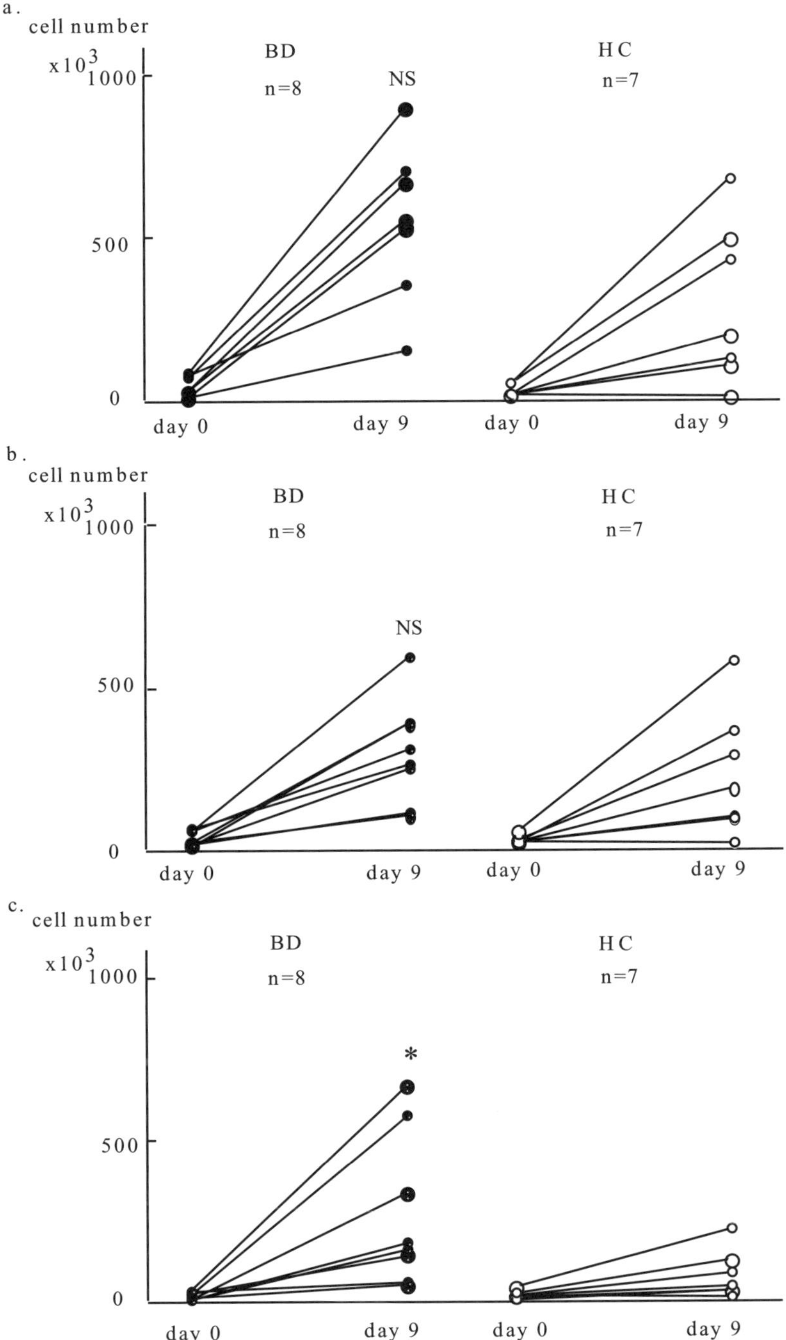

Figure 1 Change of γδ+ T absolute cell number of mononuclear cells in peripheral blood before and after *S. Sanguis* stimulation. Left panel: patients with Behçet's disease (BD). Right panel: healthy controls (HC). a. whole γδ+ T cells. b. γδ +CD4-CD8- T cells. c. γδ +CD8+ T cells (NS: no significant, *: p < 0.05).

γδ+ T cells in the peripheral blood of patients with Behçet's disease were investigated. We measured the proliferation of γδ+ T cells stimulated with the KTH-1 stain of *Streptococcus sanguis* (Fig. 1) [5]. The proliferation of γδ+ T cells from patients with Behçet's disease was higher than the γδ+ T cells from healthy controls. Particularly, CD8+ γδ+ T cells were significantly higher than the healthy controls. CD8+ γδ+ T cells are an extremely rare population in T cells, and several reports described their production of IFN-γ in an antigen specific manner [6]. Furthermore, CD8 is the surface marker of cytolytic T cells that recognize an antigen presented on MHC class I molecules. Recently, genetic susceptibility for Behçet's disease has been shown to be linked to MHC class I chain-related genes (MICA). The activation of CD8+γδ+ T cells may be associated with MICA expression.

REGULATORY T CELLS

Regulatory T cells are defined as a subpopulation of T cells that are distinct from helper and cytolytic T lymphocytes, which inhibit the activity of other T cells. Recently, it has been found that the immunosuppressive factors of aqueous humor are mediated by the induction of TGF-β producing T cells [7]. An adoptive transfer of the TGF-β-producing T cells suppressed the induction of delayed type hypersensitivity mediated by Th1 cells. Although the regulatory T cells suppressed IFN-γ production by the Th1 cells through bystander mechanisms, the regulatory T cells required antigen specific activation to function. Therefore, there is a potential to use such regulatory T cells to suppress and prevent the production of Th1 cytokines in Behçet's disease.

CONCLUSIONS

Th1 cells and CD8+γδ+ T cells are capable of having an important role in the immunopathogenesis of Behçet's disease. In addition, treatment for Behçet's disease may include therapeutic methods that activate regulatory T cells.

ACKNOWLEDGEMENTS

The authors thank Prof. Kenji Hirayama at the Institute of Tropical Medicine, Nagasaki Univ. Nagasaki, Japan and Dr. Andrew W. Taylor at the Schepens Eye Research Institute, Harvard Medical School, Boston, USA, for their instructions.

REFERENCES

1. Esin, S., Gul, A., Hodara, V., Jeddi-Tehrani, M., Dilsen, N., Konice, M., Andersson, R. and Wigzell H., *Clin. Exp. Immunol.* 107: 520–7, 1997.
2. Direskeneli, H., Eksioglu-Demiralp, E., Kibarogulu, A., Yavuz, S., Ergun, T. and Akoglu T., *Clin. Exp. Immunol.* 117: 166–70, 1999.

  Tomomi Nishida and Shigeaki Ohno

3. Frassanito, M.A., Dammacco, R., Cafforio, P. and Dammacco F., *Arthritis Rheum.* 42: 1967–74, 1999.

4. Sugi-Ikai, N., Nakazawa, M., Nakamura, S, Ohno, S. and Minami M., *Invest. Ophthalmol. Vis. Sci.* 39: 996–1004, 1998.

5. Nishida, T., Hirayama, K., Nakamura, S. and Ohno S., *Ocul. Immunol. Inflamm.* 6: 139–44, 1998.

6. Freysdottir, J., Lau, S. and Fortune F., *Clin. Exp. Immunol.* 118: 451–7, 1999.

7. Nishida, T. and Taylor A.W., *Invest. Ophthalmol. Vis. Sci.* 40: 2268–74, 1999.

KAZUNORI ONOÉ, NOBUYOSHI KITAICHI, SHIGEAKI OHNO,
CHIKAKO IWABUCHI AND KAZUYA IWABUCHI

7. NK and NK-T Cells Possibly Involved in Behçet's Disease

ABSTRACT

It has been considered that NK and NK-T cells play some roles in ocular autoimmune diseases such as Behçet's disease. In this communication, general functions of these-lymphocytes and a possible involvement of NK and/or NK-T cells in experimentally induced autoimmune uveoretinitis (EAU) are presented. Administration of anti-NK1.1 monoclonal antibodies to B10.BR mice significantly inhibited the severity of EAU induced by K2, an IRBP peptide, suggesting a proinflammtory role of NK1.1 positive lymphocytes in the EAU.

KEYWORDS   NK cells; NK-T cells; EAU; ITIM; NKR-P1(NK1.1)

INTRODUCTION

NK and NK-T cells may represent cells involved in cross-talking between innate and acquired immunities [1–3]. Thus, it seems that the NK and NK-T cells play a role in induction and/or regulation of various types of immune responses including several autoimmune diseases [4, 5]. It has been reported that certain ocular inflammations such as Behçet's disease result from organ specific autoimmune responses [6, 7]. Thus far, no concrete evidences have been presented whether NK or NK-T cells are really involved in induction or regulation of Behçet's disease and studies of the role of NK and NK-T cells in this disease are far from complete. In the present communication, general characteristics as well as possible roles of NK and NK-T cells in organ specific autoimmune diseases are presented and discussed.

NK CELLS

NK cells kill certain kind of tumor cells, virus-infected cells and target cells coated by antibodies (ADCC). NK cells also produce pro-inflammatory cytokines such as TNF-α and IFN-γ. Thus, NK cells appear to play a major role in anti-tumor immune responses and infectious immunity through the cytotoxicity and cytokine productions.

Murine NK cells express Ly 49, a lectin type receptor (Fig. 1). When Ly 49 binds to certain type major histocompatibility complex (MHC) class I molecules, an inhibitory signal is transduced intracellularly, and the NK cells no more kill the target. On the other hand, NK cells kill the target when Ly 49 is blocked by a specific antibody (Ab). NK cell also can kill the class I null cells. Figure 1 shows the most primitive framework of "missing self" hypothesis [8].

Two types of inhibitory receptors are expressed on human NK cells. NK cells express p58 killer inhibitory receptors (KIR), which belong to Ig superfamily. The p58KIR possesses immunoreceptor tyrosine-based inhibition motif (ITIM) [9] in the cytoplasmic tail (Fig. 2). When p58KIR binds to HLA-C, an inhibitory signal is induced and the NK functions inhibited.

The other inhibitory receptor is a lectin type receptor which also possesses ITIM in its cytoplasmic region. The inhibitory signal is generated when CD94 binds to HLA-E, a non-classical MHC class I molecule (Fig. 2). Interestingly, HLA-E requires binding of a nonamer peptide for cell surface expression [10]. This peptide was derived from the signal sequences of most classical HLA class I molecules. Thus, HLA-E surface expression allows NK cells to monitor the expression of numerous polymor-

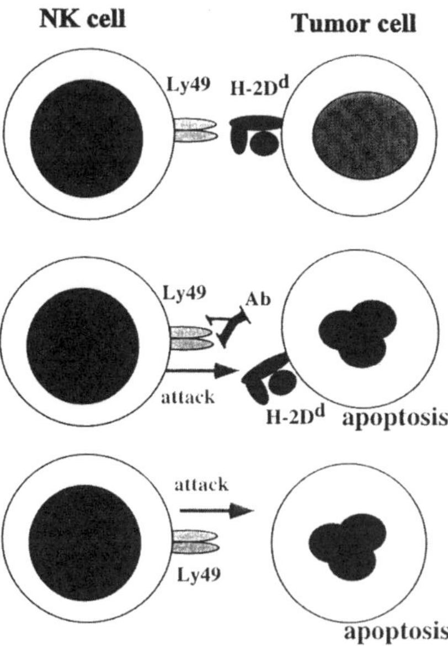

Figure 1 NK cells kill the target missing self MHC Ag.

                                                    Kazunori Onoé et al.

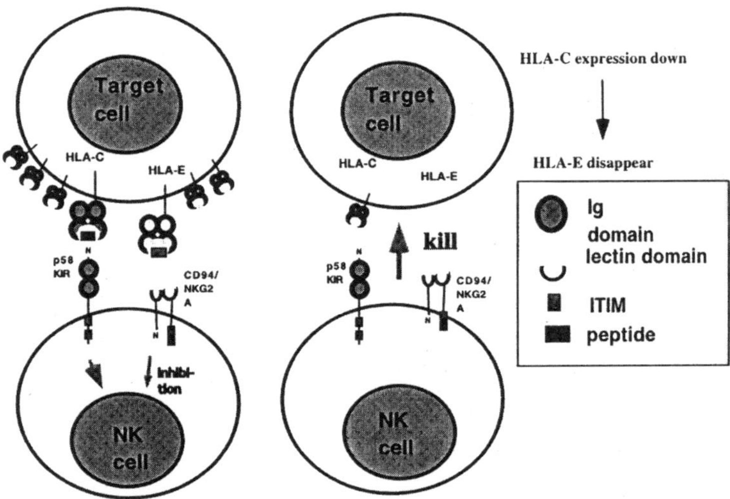

Figure 2 Two types of inhibitory receptors on NK cells.

phic HLA class I molecules with a single receptor, CD94/NKG2A. As shown in Figure 2 right panel, reduction of HLA-C molecule leads to the reduction of the signal sequences required for the expression of HLA-E. Eventually, expressions of both the HLA-C and HLA-E molecules on the target are reduced and this target is recognized by NK cell as one to be destroyed.

Now we know various receptors belonging to Ig superfamily and lectin type receptors in human and murine systems (Fig. 3). Among these receptors, those possessing ITIM in the cytoplasmic tail are inhibitory receptors. It is important that different NK cell clones express different receptors. This means that each NK cell

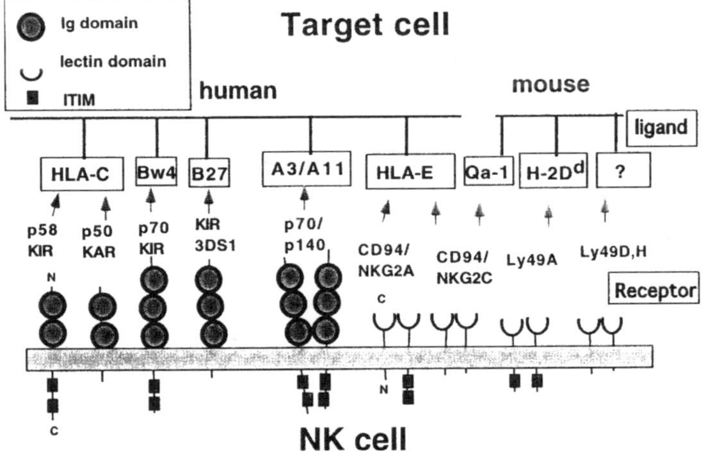

Figure 3 Various receptors on human and murine NK cells.

group shows different specificity for inhibition mediated by different MHC class I- or class I-like molecules.

NK-T CELLS

In 1987, Fowlkes et al. [11] and Ceredig et al. [12] reported a unique thymocyte population in CD4, 8 double negative cells. We found a similar population in CD4$^+$ thymocytes [13]. Now these cells are called NK-T cells or natural T cells and constitute more complex subsets including CD8$^+$ NK-T cells [14, 15]. These cells show a differentiation pattern quite different from the mainstream T cells. In the thymus NK T cells are positively selected in the presence of CD1 or TL molecules expressed on CD4$^+$8$^+$ thymocytes [16, 17]. Recently we have demonstrated that thymic medullary epithelial cells are also indispensable for the NK-T generation [18, 19]. It appears that the direct precursors of NK-T cells are NK1.1$^+$ CD3$^-$ cells that quite resemble phenotypically and functionally NK cells [20, 21].

The general characteristics of NK-T cells are summarized in Table 1. NK-T cells express both NK receptors and α/β T cell antigen (Ag) receptors (TCR) (Fig. 4). These cells phenotypically resemble memory T cells except for the expression of NK1.1 and Ly49. Thus, these are CD44$^+$, ICAM-1$^+$, LFA-1$^+$, IL-2Rβ$^+$ and CD62L$^-$. NK-T cells are relatively abundant in the thymus, bone marrow and liver but not in peripheral lymph nodes. Interestingly, certain self-reactive NK-T cells are not eliminated by negative selection [13].

We have reported that NK-T cells kill both tumor cells and self immature thymocytes [22, 23] and produce IL-4 and IFN-γ upon stimulation via TCR [24].

It has been reported that NK-T cells expressing invariant Vα (Vα14Jα281) chains recognize glycosylphosphatidyl inositol (GPI)-anchored Ag in the context of CD1, an MHC-class Ib molecule (Fig. 4) [25]. A majority of murine NK-T cells express

Table 1   Characteristics of NK-T cells.

1.	Expression of both NK cell markers (NKR-P1, Ly49) and α β/TCR
2.	Phenotypically resemble memory T cells
3.	Relatively abundant in thymus, bone marrow and liver
4.	Limited usage of α/β TCR
5.	Existence of autoreactive cells (forbidden clone)
6.	LAK activity against tumor cells and thymocytes
7.	Cytotoxicity against immature thymocytes via FasL-Fas interaction
8.	Prominent productions of IL-4 and IFN-γ

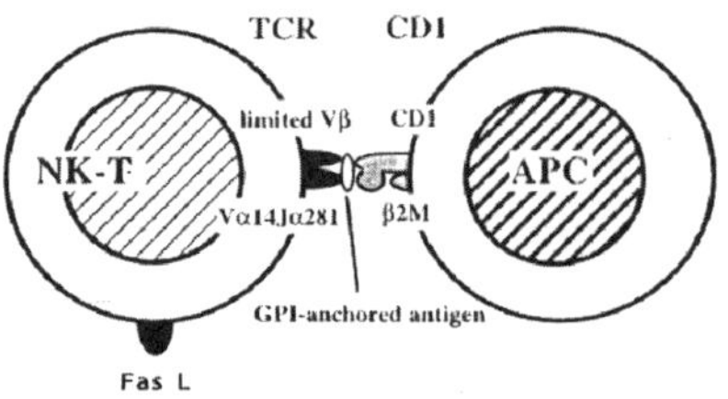

Figure 4 NK-T cell recognizes GPI-anchored Ag with CD1.

Kazunori Onoé et al.

Vα14Jα281 and Vβ8 and most of human NK-T cells express Vα24Vβ11, a counter-
part of Vα14Vβ8 in murine NK-T cells [26].

However, using TCR-transgenic mice, we and others found that functional NK-T
cells carrying the other TCR Vα chains were normally generated [27, 28]. The entire
Ag system that NK-T cells recognize has not been fully elucidated.

It seems most interesting to us that NK-T cells express constitutively FasL. In
normal mice the NK-T cells kill the self CD4, 8 double positive (DP) thymocytes
bearing Fas molecules [23] (Fig. 5). However, in *lpr* or *gld* mouse, this killing system
doesn't work. CD4, 8 DP thymocytes of *lpr* mouse express no Fas Ag because of
mutation of the *fas* gene. Thus, these DP cells can not be killed by NK-T cells. On the
other hand, NK-T cells of *gld* mouse can not kill the DP thymocytes due to the point
mutation of the FasL expressed on the *gld* NK-T cells.

In physiological conditions, most of CD4, 8 DP thymocytes undergo apoptosis and
only a few selected T cells migrate outside the thymus. However, in these *lpr* and *gld*
mice, no such a death system operates and massive proliferation of abnormal lymphocytes is seen (Fig. 6). In addition, the subsequent autoimmune disease kill these *lpr*
and *gld* mice early in life. We would like to postulate that NK-T cells in the thymus
eliminate abnormally developed lymphocytes, and by this way maintain the homeos-
tasis.

In peripheral immune system, it is also speculated that NK-T cells regulate excess
or undesirable immune responses [4, 5, 29, 30]. It will be seen in Figure 7 that a self
Ag reactive helper T cell is continuously activated with the self Ag *in vivo* and
expressing Fas molecules. Under normal conditions, this helper T cell is killed by NK-
T cells and the autoimmune responses appear to be stamped out. Indeed it was reported that the number of NK-T cell decreased in certain types of systemic autoimmune
disease in animal models and human cases [31, 32].

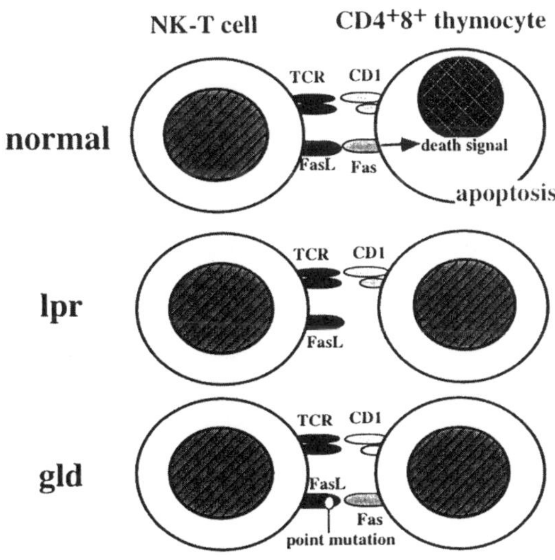

Figure 5 NK-T cell kills CD4, 8 DP thymocytes via Fas.

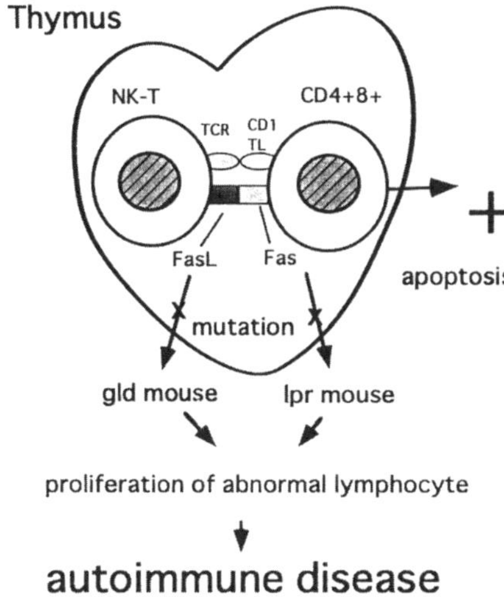

Figure 6 Lack of NK-T functions results in auto-immune disease in *lpr* and *gld* mice.

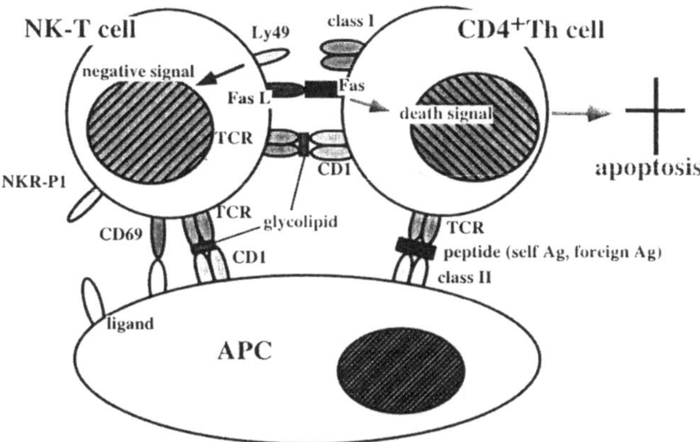

Figure 7 NK-T cell may kill self-reactive Th cell.

These decreases may be related to the insufficient regulation of immune responses to the self Ag by NK-T cells.

ROLES OF NK AND/OR NK-T CELLS IN EXPERIMENTALLY INDUCED AUTOIMMUNE UVEORETINITIS (EAU), AN EXPERIMENTAL MODEL OF BEHÇET'S DISEASE

We postulated that NK-T cells also played a regulatory role in experimental autoimmune uveoretinitis (EAU), a model for Behçet's disease. To examine this working hypothesis, we performed the following experiment.

                                                     Kazunori Onoé et al.

We have reported that a peptide, K2, deduced from interphotoreceptor retinoid-binding protein (IRBP) induces EAU in H-2^k mice [33, 34]. Using this model we examined our hypothesis that NK-T cells regulate EAU by eliminating the K2-specific T cells. H-2^k mice were administrated anti-NK1.1 Ab and immunized with K2 in complete Freund's adjuvant. Thereafter T cell responses to K2 peptides and clinical manifestation of EAU were examined (Fig. 8).

Figure 9 shows a representative result of T cell proliferative responses to K2 10 days after immunization. As shown in this figure, however, treatment with anti-NK1.1 Ab exerted no influence on the T cell responses.

In addition, anti-NK1.1 Ab treatment rather reduced the clinical severity of EAU (Fig. 10). Since this Ab treatment eliminates both NK and NK-T cell populations, it seems difficult to draw a straightforward interpretation from this preliminary experiment. Thus far, our study suggests that NK and/or NK-T cells may enhance the local inflammation rather than negative regulation.

Recently it was reported that the number of CD56$^+$ T cells increased in patients with Behçet's disease [35].

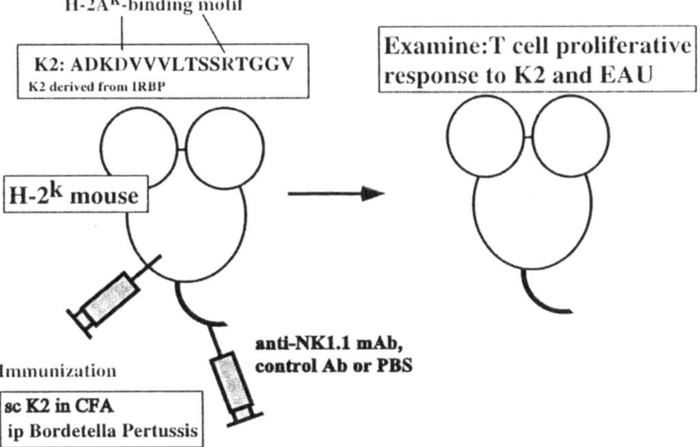

Figure 8 Experimental procedure to examine influence of eradication of NK1.1$^+$ cells on EAU.

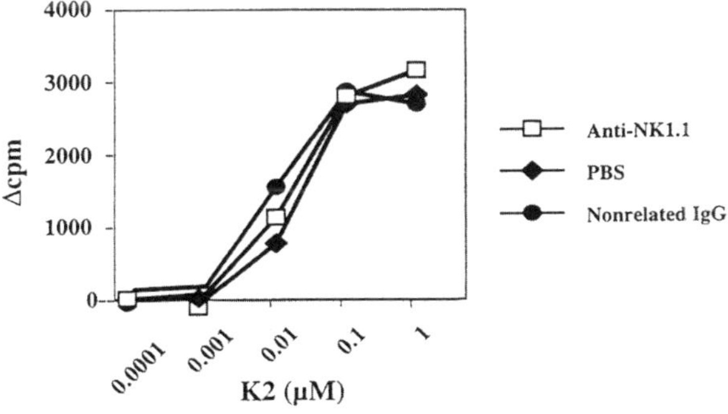

Figure 9 T cell proliferative response to K2.

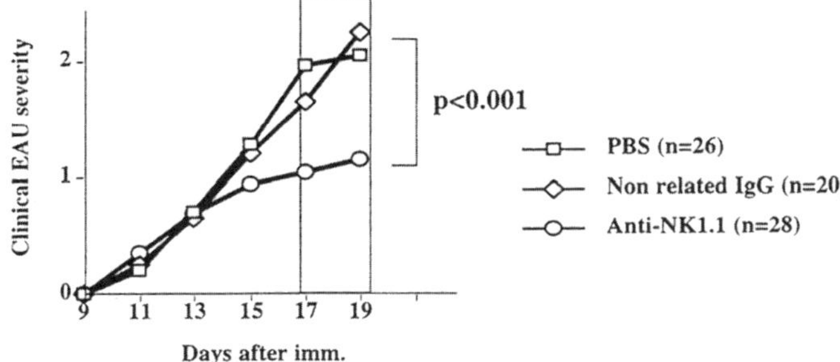

Fig. 10   Time course of clinical EAU.

Although CD56$^+$ T cells are not necessarily corresponding to NK-T cells, this result appears to be consistent with our experiment. In addition, we reported that activated NK-T cells expressed mRNA of macrophage migration inhibitory factor (MIF) [36]. Thus, it seems that NK T cells produce MIF other than IL-4 and IFNγ. Administration of anti-MIF Ab inhibited R16, a peptide deduced from IRBP, – induced EAU in a rat system [37]. Indeed, serum MIF levels in patients with Behçet's disease were prominently increased [38]. These series of study also suggest that NK-T cells enhance ocular inflammation via cytokine productions. More precise studies of patients with Behçet's disease are needed to see how NK and NK-T cells and cytokines produced by NK-T cells are involved in the ocular inflammatory disease.

CONCLUSION

General characteristics of NK and NK-T cells and their possible involvement in EAU, an experimental model for Behçet's disease, are discussed. It appears that NK1.1$^+$ cells rather enhance ocular inflammatory responses. However, the study is just beginning and experimentation in which specific elimination of NK-T population *in vivo* is performed appears to be needed. We are now carrying out EAU experiment in NK-T knockout mice to elucidate the precise role of NK-T cells.

ACKNOWLEDGMENTS

We thank Ms Kaori Kohno for her secretarial assistance. This study was supported in part by a Grant-in-Aid from Ministry of Education, Science, Sports and Culture, Japan.

REFERENCES

1. Eberl. G., Brawand, P. and MacDonald, R., *J. Immunol.*, 165: 4305–4311, 2000.
2. Tomomura, M., Yu, W.-G., Ahn, H.-J., Yamashita, M., Yang, Y.-F., Ono, S., Hamaoka, T., Kawano, T., Taniguchi, M., Koezuka, Y. and Fujiwara, H., *J. Immunol.*, 163: 93–101, 1999.

                                                                 Kazunori Onoé et al.

3. Carmaud, C., Lee, D., Donnars, O., Park, S-H., Beavis, A., Kozuka, Y. and Bendelac, A., *J. Immunol.*, 163: 4647–4650, 1999.

4. Sonoda, K., Exley, M., Snapper, S., Balk, S. P. and Stein-Streilein, *J. Exp. Med.*, 190: 1215–1225, 1999.

5. Hammond, K.J.H., Poulton, L.D., Palmisano, L.J., Silveira, P.A. Godfrey, D.I. and Baxter, A. G., *J. Exp. Med.*, 187: 1047–1056, 1998.

6. Terrant, T.K., Silver, P.B., Wahlsten, J.L., Rizzo, L.V., Chan, C-C., Wiggert, B. and Caspi, R. R., *J. Exp. Med.*, 189: 219–230, 1999.

7. Sun, B., Sun, S.-H., Chan, C.-C., Wiggert, B. and Caspi, R.R., *Int. Immunol.*, 11: 1307–1312, 1999.

8. Ljunggren, H.-G. and Kärre, K., *Immunol. Today*, 11: 237–244, 1990.

9. Isakov, N., *Adv. Immunol.*, 69: 183–247, 1998.

10. Tomsec, P., Braud, V. M., Rikards, C., Powell, M.B., McSharry, B.P., Gadola, S., Cerundolo, V., Borysiewicz, L.K., McMichael, A.J. and Wilkinson, G.W.G., *Science*, 287: 1031–1033, 2000.

11. Fowlkes, B.J., Kruisbeek, A.M., That, H.T., Weston, M.A., Coligan, J.E., Schwartz, R.H. and Pardoll, D.M., *Nature*, 329: 251–253, 1987.

12. Ceredig, R., Lynch, F. and Newman, P., *Proc. Natl. Acad. Sci. USA.*, 84: 8578–8582, 1987.

13. Arase, H., Arase, N., Ogasawara, K., Good, R.A. and Onoé, K., *Proc. Natl. Acad. Sci. USA.*, 89: 6506–6510, 1992.

14. Emoto, M., Zerrahn, J., Miyamoto, M., Pérarnau, B. and Kaufman, S.H.H., *Eur. J. Immunol.*, 30: 2300–2311, 2000.

15. Apostolou, I., Cumano, A., Gachelin, G. and Kourilsky, P., *J. Immunol.* 165: 2481–2490, 2000.

16. Bendelac, A., *Curr. Opin. Immunol.*, 7: 367–374, 1995.

17. MacDonald, R., *J. Exp. Med.*, 182: 633–638, 1995.

18. Nakagawa, K., Iwabuchi, K., Ogasawara, K., Ato, M., Kajiwara, M., Nishihori, H., Iwabuchi, C., Ishikawa, H., Good, R.A. and Onoé, K., *Proc. Natl. Acad. Sci. USA.*, 94: 2472–2477, 1997.

19. Konishi, J., Iwabuchi, K., Iwabuchi, C., Ato, M., Nagata, J., Onoé, K.Jr., Nakagawa, K., Kasai, M., Ogasawara, K., Kawakami, K. and Onoé, K., *Cell. Immunol.*, 206: 26–35, 2000.

20. Tone, S., Iwabuchi, K., Iwabuchi, C., Negishi, I. and Onoé, K., *Immunol. Lett.*, 73: 65–69, 2000.

21. Iwabuchi, K., Iwabuchi, C., Tone, S., Itoh, D., Tosa, N., Negishi, I., Ogasawara, K., Uede, T. and Onoé, K., *Blood*, 97: 1765–1775, 2001.

22. Arase, H., Arase-Fukushi, N., Good, R.A. and Onoé, K., *J. Immunol.*, 151: 546–555, 1993.

23. Arase, H., Arase, N., Kobayashi, Y., Nishimura, Y., Yonehara, S. and Onoé, K., *J. Exp. Med.*, 180: 423–432, 1994.

24. Arase, H., Arase, N., Nakagawa, K., Good, R.A. and Onoé, K., *Eur. J. Immunol.*, 23: 307–310, 1993.

25. Schofield, L., McConville, M.J., Hansen, D., Campbell, A.S., Fraser-Reid, B., Grusby, M. J. and Tachado, S.D., *Science*, 283: 225–229, 1999.

26. Prussin, C. and Foster, B., *J. Immunol.*, 159: 5862–5870, 1997.

27. Iwabuchi, C., Iwabuchi, K., Nakagawa, K., Takayanagi, T., Nishihori, H., Tone, S., Ogasawara, K., Good, R.A. and Onoé, K., *Proc. Natl. Acad. Sci. USA.*, 95: 8199–8204, 1998.

28. Schultz, R. -J., Parkes, A., Mizoguchi, E., Bhan, A. and Koyasu, S., *J. Immunol.*, 157: 4379–4389, 1996.

29. Singh, N., Hong, S., Scherer, D.C., Serizawa, I., Burdin, N., Kronenberg, M., Kozuka, Y. and Kaer, L.V., *J. Immunol.*, 163: 2373–2377, 1999.

30. Lehuen, A., Lants, O., Beaudoin, L., Laloux, V., Carnaud, C., Bendelac, A., Bach, J.-F. and Monteiro, R.C., *J. Exp. Med.*, 188: 1831–1839, 1998

31. Mieza, M.A., Itoh, T., Cui, J.Q., Makino, Y., Kawano, T., Tsuchida, K., Koike, T., Shirai, T., Yagita, H., Matsuzawa, A., Koseki, H. and Taniguchi, M., *J. Immunol.*, 156: 4035–4040, 1996.

32. Sumida, T., Sakamoto, A., Murata, H., Makino, Y., Takahashi, H., Yoshida, S., Nishioka, K., Iwamoto, I. and Tainiguchi, M., *J. Exp. Med.*, 182: 1163–1168, 1995.

33. Namba, K., Ogasawara, K., Kitaichi, N., Matsuki, N., Takahashi, A., Sasamoto, Y., Kotake, S., Matsuda, H., Iwabuchi, K., Ohno, S. and Onoé, K., *Clin. Exp. Immunol.*, 111: 442–449, 1998.

34. Namba, K., Ogasawara, K., Kitaichi, N., Morohashi, T., Sasamoto, Y., Kotake, S., Matsuda, H., Iwabuchi, K., Iwabuchi, C., Ohno, S. and Onoé, K., *J. Immunol.*, 65: 2962–2969, 2000.

35. Yato, H. and Matsumoto, Y., *Br.J. Ophthalmol.*, 83: 1386–1389, 1999.

36. Kitaichi, N., Ogasawara, K., Iwabuchi, K., Nishihira, J., Namba, K., Onoé, K.Jr., Konishi, J., Kotake, S., Matsuda, H. and Onoé, K., *Immunobiol.*, 201: 356–367, 2000.

37. Kitaichi, N., Matsuda, A., Kotake, S., Namba, K., Tagawa, Y., Sasamoto, Y., Ogasawara, K., Iwabuchi, K., Onoé, K., Matsuda, H. and Nishihira, J., *Curr. Eye Res.*, 20: 109–114. 2000.

38. Kitaichi, N., Kotake, S., Sasamoto, Y., Namba, K., Matsuda, A., Ogasawara, K., Onoé, K., Matsuda, H. and Nishihira, J., *Invest. Ophtalmol. Vis. Sci.*, 40: 247–250, 1999.

Kazunori Onoé et al.

AHMET GÜL

8. Cytokines in Behçet's Disease

ABSTRACT

The aetiopathogenesis of Behçet's disease is unknown, but studies indicate that various immunological abnormalities, induced by certain microbial antigens in genetically susceptible individuals, play an important role in the development of Behçet's disease.

Immunological studies in Behçet's disease have revealed *in vivo* activation of T cells (both TCR $\alpha\beta$ and $\gamma\delta$ positive), natural killer cells, monocytes and neutrophils in parallel with up-regulated proinflammatory cytokines. Expression of IL-12 and IL-8 cytokines and Th1 polarization of the immune response are associated with the active disease. However, no prominent increase of Th2 cytokines has been detected with decreasing clinical activity.

The enhanced expression of proinflammatory and Th1-type cytokines suggests a defect in the regulatory mechanisms; and it may have a genetic basis. But, no strong association could be documented between cytokine gene polymorphisms and Behçet's disease so far.

We still need more data about the characteristics of cytokine expression in Behçet's disease to develop better and more targeted treatment modalities.

KEYWORDS: Behçet's disease; cytokines; Th1 polarization; proinflammatory cytokines; cytokine antagonists; cytokine gene polymorphisms; tumour necrosis factor; interleukin-8; interleukin-12

INTRODUCTION

Behçet's disease is a chronic inflammatory disorder characterized by recurrent attacks of different clinical manifestations, including oral aphthous ulcers, genital ulcers, uveitis, skin lesions, arthritis, venous thrombosis, arterial aneurysms, and lesions in the central nervous and gastrointestinal systems [1]. It is recognized as an unclassified form of systemic vasculitis, which affects almost all types and sizes of blood vessels.

The aetiopathogenesis of Behçet's disease is unknown, but studies indicate a multifactorial disorder. It has long been claimed that various immunological abnormalities, induced by certain microbial antigens in genetically susceptible individuals, play an important role in the development of Behçet's disease [2]. The immunological studies have revealed an enhanced inflammatory response, with findings of non-specific activation of many different inflammatory cells as well as antigen-driven specific immune response. Thus, immune-mediated inflammatory reaction of Behçet's disease involves both innate and adaptive immune systems [2].

Cytokines are important small molecules acting as short-range intercellular messengers, and they play a crucial role in inflammatory reactions. Cytokines are produced by a wide variety of cells to be effective mainly in a microenvironment, and they bind specific receptors on the cell surface to induce many different functions. Their activity is tightly controlled by various ways, including transcriptional and post-transctiptional mechanisms, or by through soluble receptors and receptor antagonists. Cytokines also show promoting or antagonistic effects on each other and provide a balanced immune response [3]. Th1 type cytokines, such as interleukin (IL)-2 and interferon (IFN)-γ promote development of T cells expressing similar cytokines, and also supress the production of Th2 type cytokines, such as IL-4 and IL-10. On the other hand, IL-4 enhances the development of Th2 cells and down-regulates differentiation into or activation of Th1 cells. Defects in these control mechanisms have been suggested as one of the important components of the subacute or chronic inflammatory conditions.

Understanding the nature of inflammation in Behçet's disease by the analysis of the cytokine network is very important for the clarification of the disease pathogenesis. Successful results using cytokines (such as IFN-α) or cytokine antagonists (anti-tumour necrosis factor-α [TNF-α] monoclonal antibody) in the treatment of Behçet's disease also make this analysis necessary for developing better treatment modalities, which target more specific inflammatory mediators.

Cytokine studies in Behçet's disease have mainly been carried out in systemic circulation or in supernatants of peripheral blood mononuclear cell cultures. More recently, investigation of intracytoplasmic cytokine expression patterns in isolated cells has enabled us to see a better picture of the cytokine network in Behçet's disease.

SYSTEMIC CIRCULATION

Increased or detectable serum/plasma levels of TNF-α, IFN-γ, IL-1, IL-8, IL-10 , IL-12, soluble IL-2 receptor (sIL-2R) and 75 kD TNF receptor (TNFR-75) were reported in Behçet's disease [4–16]. An increase in the levels of IL-8, IL-12, sIL-2R and TNFR-75 was detected in the active stage of patients with Behçet's disease [10–16]. However, lymphocyte derived IFN-γ was found only in the sera of inactive patients [4].

On the other hand, some investigators did not find any difference between the serum levels of TNF-α, IFN-γ, IL-1, IL-4, IL-6, IL-8, IL-10, IL-12 and transforming growth factor (TGF)-β1 in patients with Behçet's and healthy controls, or could not detect these cytokines at all [6,9,10,15,17–20].

Inconsistent results of serum cytokine concentrations in Behçet's disease can easily be explained by biological and/or technical factors. Although Behçet's disease is a multi-system disease, it is characterized with recurrent attacks of one or a combination of its clinical manifestations. Depending on the extent and severity of clinical manifestations, systemic inflammatory response is not a frequent feature of Behçet's disease. No well-defined correlation have been detected between the disease activity and acute phase response in Behçet's disease. Cytokines are effective mainly at the site of inflammation with a very short half-life, and systemic levels of many cytokines do not reflect their local activity. Circulating cytokine inhibitors such as soluble receptors and/or receptor antagonists also influence their serum levels. On the other hand, using different detection methods with varying sensitivities as well as blood collection and storage conditions could also have contributed to these inconsistent results.

CELL CULTURE ASSAYS

Analysis of cytokine expression in a heterogenous population of PBMC or isolated populations of monocytes or T cells in *in vitro* conditions has been accepted as a better way of investigation, and gives us a more detailed information about the cytokine kinetics in Behçet's disease. However, the cell culture assays have also many drawbacks, which should be kept in mind when comparing the results of different studies. Despite the local nature of inflammation, these studies have mostly been done using peripheral blood cells. In addition, mixed or isolated cell populations have been stimulated by using different means (such as phytohaemaglutinin, phorbol myristate acetate with ionomycin, anti-CD3, anti-CD40, various bacterial antigens or specific peptides) with varying incubation times.

Mege et al. investigated the cytokine production from Behçet's disease monocytes and detected a spontaneous over-production of TNF-α, IL-6 and IL-8 in the supernatant of monocyte cultures in active patients. An increased production of TNF-α, IL-1, IL-6 and IL-8 from monocytes was also observed with lipopolysaccharide (LPS) stimulation in both inactive and active patients [21].

IL-2 production from lymphocytes following mitogen-stimulation was found to be normal or increased in Behçet's disease [22]. However, concanavalin A (Con A)-activated T cells failed to proliferate normally in response to exogenous IL-2 stimulation, regardless of the disease activity of the patients. This unresponsiveness of T cells to IL-2 was explained by a substantial decrease in the number of cells bearing high affinity IL-2R in active patients with Behçet's disease, and a decrease in the relative numbers of receptors on the IL-2R positive T cells in inactive and chronic active patients [22,23].

Intracytoplasmic cytokine expression of individual cells by flow cytometry revealed increased percentage of IL-2 and IFN-γ producing T cells in active patients with Behçet's disease [16,24]. High serum levels of IL-12 in parallel with an increased frequency of peripheral IL-2 and IFN-γ producing T cells suggested a strong, polarized Th1 immune response in vivo [16]. A decrease of Th1 type T cells was found following the immunosuppressive treatment of active patients. However, no increase in Th2 type IL-4 producing T cells was observed during inactive stage of patients with

Behçet's disease [16,24]. Suzuki and colleagues' findings of up-regulated expression of IL-12 receptor β chain and transcription factor Txk in T cells further supported a Th1 polarized immune response in Behçet's disease (N. Suzuki, personal communication).

T cell lines from pustular skin lesions of 4 patients were established using a streptococcal antigen KTH-1. Two of these cell lines were CD8$^+$TCR αβ$^+$ and expressed IL-8 and TNF-α mRNAs. Other cell lines were CD4$^+$TCR αβ$^+$, and 1 of them expressed Th1, the other one Th2 cytokines [25].

Analysis of γδ T cell populations also revealed that significantly increased proportion of γδ T cells were in the activated stage and producing both IFN-γ and TNF-α [26,27]. In contrast to the αβ T cells, CD25 (the α chain of IL-2R) expression on γδ T cells was found to be increased. Yamashita et al. reported that CD45RA$^+$ γδ T cells produced more TNF-α and lymphotoxin-α (LT-α) than CD45RO$^+$ γδ T cells, while both subsets were producing equal amounts of IL-8, but no IL-4 at all [28].

Stimulation of PBMC from Behçet's disease patients with specific human 60-kD heat shock protein (hsp)-derived peptide 336–351 induced the expression of proinflammatory cytokine mRNAs, including IL-8, TNF-α, LT-α [29]. Hirohata et al showed that this hypersensitivity of T cells in Behçet's disease is not restricted to the disease specific hsp peptides, and low concentrations of staphylococcal enterotoxins could stimulate Behçet's disease T cells through T cell receptor β chain for IFN-γ production much more effectively than normal or rheumatoid arthritis T cells [30].

It was recently demonstrated that neutrophils from patients with Behçet's disease constitutively expressed TNF-α mRNA and produced increased amounts of TNF-α with LPS stimulation [31,32]. Neutrophils in Behçet's disease also produced IL-12 and IL-18 spontaneously, which suggest that these activated neutrophils might play a role in the Th1 polarization of the immune response [31,32].

TISSUE EXPRESSION

There are very limited published data on the cytokine expression of infiltrating cells at the site of inflammation in Behçet's disease. Kikkawa et al. reported expression of IFN-γ and IL-6 in the dermal and perivascular infiltrates in the erythema nodosumlike lesions [33]. They also detected perivascular IL-8 in the deep dermis and interlipocellular areas of the erythema-nodosum like lesions, as well as in an oral aphthous ulcer [33]. Freysdottir and colleagues analysed the intracellular and membrane-bound cytokines in the oral aphthous ulcer lesions of patients with Behçet's disease, and found an abundant infiltration of TNF-α positive cells that extend into the submucosa [34].

GENETIC POLYMORPHISMS

Genetic polymorphisms in the promoter, coding and/or 3'-untranslated regions have been suggested to influence the expression of many cytokines. Polymorphisms in the TNF-α and LT-α genes have been investigated thoroughly in Behçet's disease because of the close proximity of these genes to HLA-B. Behçet's disease is strongly associated with HLA-B51, and it has been hypothesized that polymorphisms in the TNF genes might contribute to the pathogenesis of Behçet's disease [35]. The 10.5 kB allele (TNFB*2) of bi-allelic *Nco* I digestion polymorphism in the LT-α gene has been shown to be in linkage disequilibrium with a number of HLA-B alleles, including HLA-B51 [36]. An increase of TNFB*2 in parallel with the decrease of 5,5 kB (TNFB*1) allele was observed in Behçet's disease patients, especially in those with severe ocular involvement [36,37]. This association is not stronger than that of HLA-B51 with Behçet's disease, but it is difficult to assess the individual contribution of these polymorphisms in the neighbouring genes, which are co-inherited with HLA-B51 on the same haplotype, to the disease pathogenesis.

The rare allele (TNF2) of the promoter region $-308G{\rightarrow}A$ polymorphism in the TNF-α gene, has been shown to be associated with increased TNF-α expression, and is in linkage disequilibrium with the extended haplotype of HLA-A1-B8-DR3-DQ2 [38]. No association could be detected between TNF2 allele and Behçet's disease [37,39]. We could not demonstrate any association of the TNF-α -376 polymorphism with Behçet's disease either (J. Duymaz, unpublished).

We have recently identified a modest association of IL-1A gene polymorphism with Behçet's disease (J. Karasneh, unpublished). However, no significant result was obtained in the association studies with IL-6 and IL-8 genes, both of which have been shown to be over-expressed in Behçet's disease [40], (J. Duymaz, unpublished).

Further studies, especially on the posttranscriptional regulatory mechanisms, are still needed for the identification of the contributory role of genetic polymorphisms to the susceptibility to Behçet's disease.

EXPERIMENTAL MODELS

Despite several attempts, there is no established animal model for Behçet's disease. None of the clinical findings of Behçet's disease were observed in the HLA-B51 transgenic mice [41]. After the identification of Behçet's disease-specific hsp-peptides, uveitogenic features of these peptides were documented in Lewis rats [42]. However, these animals did not develop any other Behçet's disease-related manifestations. It was recently demonstrated that mucosal administration of these hsp-peptides can also induce uveitis [43]. Although, CD4+ T cells were the main effector cells in the induction of hsp uveitis, investigation of CD4-enriched splenic cells by reverse transcription-PCR did not reveal any significant difference in the expression of Th1 or Th2 cytokines. However, treatment with exogenous IL-4 significantly decreased the development of uveitis induced by mucosal administration of hsp peptide 336–351 from 68% to 30.4% [43].

Sohn and colleagues described another animal model induced by inoculation of herpes simplex virus type I to the ICR mice [44]. About 30% of these mice developed various manifestations, some of which resembling to those of Behçet's disease. The authors recently reported that up-regulated Th2 cytokines can attenuate the development of the skin manifestations in the ICR model [45].

Unfortunately, both of these animal models are far from answering the questions in the pathogenesis of Behçet's disease, especially about the therapeutic use of cytokines and/or cytokine antagonists.

CONCLUSIONS

In conclusion, immunological studies in Behçet's disease have revealed *in vivo* activation of T cells (both TCR αβ and γδ positive), natural killer cells, monocytes and neutrophils in parallel with up-regulated proinflammatory cytokines. Expression of IL-12 and IL-8 cytokines and Th1 polarization of the immune response are associated with the active disease. However, no prominent increase of Th2 cytokines has been detected with decreasing clinical activity.

The enhanced expression of proinflammatory cytokines suggests a defect in the regulatory mechanisms, and it may have a genetic basis. But, no strong association could be documented between a cytokine gene polymorphism and Behçet's disease so far.

We still need more data about the characteristics of cytokine expression in Behçet's disease to develop better and more targeted treatment modalities.

REFERENCES

1. Sakane, T., Takeno, M., Suzuki, N. and Inaba, G., *N. Engl. J. Med.* 341: 1284–1291, 1999.
2. Gül, A., *Clin. Exp. Rheumatol.* 2001 (in press).
3. Abbas, A.K., Murphy, K.M. and Sher, A, *Nature* 383: 787–793, 1996.
4. Fujii, N., Minagawa, T., Nakane, A., Kato, F. and Ohno, S., *J. Immunol.* 130: 1683–6, 1983.
5. Hamzaoui, K., Ayed, K., Slim, A., Hamza, M. and Touraine, J., *Clin. Exp. Immunol.* 79: 28–34, 1990.
6. Hamzaoui, K., Hamza, M., and Ayed, K., *J. Rheumatol.* 17: 1428–1429, 1990.
7. Akoglu, T., Direskeneli, H., Yazici, H. and Lawrence, R., *J. Rheumatol.* 17: 1107–1108, 1990.
8. Yosipovitch, G., Shohat, B., Bshara, J., Wysenbeek, A. and Weinberger, A., *Isr. J. Med. Sci.* 31: 345–348, 1995.
9. Sayinalp, N., Ozcebe, O.I., Ozdemir, O., Haznedaroglu, I.C., Dundar, S. and Kirazli, S., *J. Rheumatol.* 23: 321–322, 1996.
10. Al-Dalaan, A., Al-Sedairy, S., Al-Balaa, S., et al., *J. Rheumatol.* 22: 904–907, 1995.
11. Sahin, S., Akoglu, T., Direskeneli, H., Sen, L.S. and Lawrence, R., *Ann. Rheum. Dis.* 55: 128–133, 1996.
12. Katsantonis, J., Adler, Y., Orfanos, C.E. and Zouboulis, C.C., *Dermatology* 201: 37–39, 2000.
13. Zouboulis, C.C., Katsantonis, J., Ketteler, R., et al., *Arch. Dermatol. Res.* 292: 279–284, 2000.
14. Hamzaoui, K. and Ayed, K.H., *J. Rheumatol.* 16: 852, 1989.
15. Turan, B., Gallati, H., Erdi, H., Gürler, A., Michel, B.A. and Villiger, P.M., *J. Rheumatol.* 24: 128–132, 1997.
16. Frassanito, M.A., Dammacco, R., Cafforio, P. and Dammacco, F., *Arthritis Rheum.* 42:1967–1974, 1999.

Ahmet Gül

17. Bacon, T.H., Ozbakir, F., Elms, C.A. and Denman, A.M., *Clin. Exp. Immunol.* 58: 541–547, 1984.

18. Ozoran, K., Aydintug, O., Tokgoz, G., Duzgun, N. and Tutkak, H., *Ann. Rheum. Dis.* 54: 610, 1995.

19. Mantas, C., Direskeneli, H., Eksioglu-Demiralp, E. and Akoglu, T., *J. Rheumatol.* 26: 510–512, 1999.

20. Eksioglu-Demiralp, E., Direskeneli, H. and Akoglu, T., *J. Immunol.* 24: 1010–1011, 1999.

21. Mege, J.-L., Dilsen, N., Sanguedolce, V., et al., *J. Rheumatol.* 20: 1544–1549, 1993.

22. Sakane, T., Suzuki, N., Ueda, Y., Takada, S., Murakawa, Y., Hoshino, T., Niwa, Y. and Tsunematsu, T., *Arthritis Rheum.* 29: 371–378, 1986.

23. Hamzaoui, K. and Ayed, K., *Clin. Exp. Rheum.* 8: 100–1, 1990.

24. Sugi-Ikai, N., Nakazawa, M., Nakamura, S., Ohno, S. and Minami, M., *Invest. Ophthalmol. Vis. Sci.* 39: 996–1004, 1998.

25. Mochizuki, M., Morita, E., Yamamoto, S. and Yamana, S., *J. Dermatol. Sci.* 15: 9–13, 1997.

26. Freysdottir, J., Lau, S.-H. and Fortune, F., *Clin. Exp. Immunol.* 188: 451–457, 1999.

27. Mochizuki, M., Suzuki, N., Takeno, M., et al., *Eur. J. Immunol.* 24: 1536–1543, 1994.

28. Yamashita, N., Kaneoka, H., Kaneko, S., et al., *Clin. Exp. Immunol.* 107: 241–247, 1997.

29. Kaneko, S., Suzuki, N., Yamashita, N., et al., *Clin. Exp. Immunol.* 108: 204–12, 1997.

30. Hirohata, S. and Hashimoto, S., *Clin. Exp. Immunol.* 112: 317–324, 1998.

31. Sakane, T., Suzuki, N. and Takeno, M. *8th International Congress on Behçet's Disease, Program and Abstracts*, pp. 56, Reggio Emilia, Italy, 1998.

32. Takeno, M., Shimoyama, Y., Suzuki, N. and Sakane, T., *8th International Congress on Behçet's Disease, Program and Abstracts*, p. 57, Reggio Emilia, Italy, 1998.

33. Kikkawa, Y., Maruyama, K., Iwatsuki, K. and Kaneko, F. in *Behçet's disease*, Godeau, P., Wechsler, B. (eds), pp. 45–48, Elsevier, Amsterdam, 1993.

34. Freysdottir, J., Farmer, I., Lau, S.-H., Hussain, L., Verity, D., Madanat, E., Stanford, M. and Fortune, F., *8th International Congress on Behçet's Disease, Program and Abstracts*, p. 143, Reggio Emilia, Italy, 1998.

35. Mizuki, M., Ohno, S., Sato, T., et al., *Hum. Immunol.*, 43: 129–135, 1995.

36. Mizuki, N., Inoko, H., Sugimura, K., et al., *Invest. Ophthalmol. Vis. Sci.* 33: 3084–3090, 1992.

37. Verity, D.H., Wallace, G.R., Vaughan, R.W., et al., *Tissue Antigens*, 54: 264–272, 1999.

38. Wilson, A.G., Symons, J.A., McDowell, T.L., McDevitt, H.O. and Duff, G.W., *Proc. Natl. Acad. Sci. USA*, 94: 3195–3199, 1997.

39. Duymaz, J., Gül, A., Uyar, F.A., Özbek, U. and Saruhan-Direskeneli, G., *Yonsei Med. J.*, 41 (Suppl.): 34, 2000.

40. Gül, A., Hajeer, A.H., Karasneh, J., Uyar, F.A., Saruhan, G., Ollier, W.E.R. and Silman, A., *Yonsei Med. J.*, 41 (Suppl.): 14, 2000.

41. Takeno, M., Kariyone, A., Yamashita N., et al., *Arthritis. Rheum.*, 38: 426–433, 1995.

42. Stanford, M.R., Kasp, E., Whiston, R., et al., *Clin. Exp. Immunol.*, 97: 226–231, 1994.

43. Hu, W., Hasan, A., Wilson, A., et al., *Eur. J. Immunol.*, 28: 2444–2455, 1998.

44. Sohn, S., Lee, E.S., Bang, D. and Lee, S., *Eur. J. Dermatol.*, 8: 21–23, 1998.

45. Sohn, S., Lee, E.S., Kwon, H.J., Lee, S.I., Bang, D. and Lee, S., *J. Infect. Dis.*, 183: 1180–1186, 2001.

NOBORU SUZUKI, MITSUHIRO TAKENO, YUKO TAKEBA, HIROKO
NAGAFUCHI AND TSUYOSHI SAKANE

9. Autoimmunity in Behçet's Disease

ABSTRACT

Autoimmune responses are implicated in the pathogenesis of Behçet's disease (BD).
We recently found that the peptide 336–351 of human heat shock protein 60, termed
Hu-18, provoked vigorous proliferation of T cells from BD patients in Japan, especially those having uveitis. The epitope is specific for BD, because no significant response
was detected in patients with RA and normal controls. Characterization of T cell
receptor (TCR) usage revealed that T cells expressing particular V beta subfamily
were selectively increased in response to Hu-18 stimulation in BD patients. The oligoclonal expansion of Hu-18 specific T cells becomes evident in clinical exacerbation, while it disappears during remission. The same T cell clones were re-expanded
in another clinical attack, suggesting the direct involvement of anti-Hu-18 specific T
cells in the pathogenesis of BD. The anti-Hu-18 specific T cells were categorized as
Th1 cells, because of their cytokine production profile. IL-12 receptor (IL-12R) expressing T cells, which had a high IFN-gamma producing potential, were increased in
PBL from BD patients with active disease. These data suggest that IL-12/IL-12R
system plays a vital role of Th1 polarization during active phase in BD patients. Txk,
a member of Tec tyrosine kinase family, is selectively expressed on Th1 and Th0 cells,
but not Th2 cells. Txk acts as a transcription factor specific for Th1 T cells. In
concordant with Th1 polarization in BD, circulating and tissue infiltrating T cells from
the patients expressed abundant Txk protein. Reduction of Txk expression in T cells
may lead to the correction of Th1/Th2 imbalance and disease remission in BD. Thus
Txk may become a possible therapeutic target in BD.

KEYWORDS: Heat shock protein HSP; autoimmune responses; anti-HSP immune
responses; Txk

INTRODUCTION

Autoimmune responses are implicated in the pathogenesis of Behçet's disease (BD). We have demonstrated various abnormal immune responses similar to certain autoimmune diseases in patients with BD; suppressor T cell dysfunction, defective interleukin (IL)-2 production, and polyclonal B cell activation [1–3]. Aberrant immune responses to self-antigens such as oral mucosa and skin homogenates have suggested involvement of autoimmune mechanisms in the pathogenesis of BD [4].

Microbial infection was considered as one of etiologic factors of BD. Herpes simplex virus (HSV) specific DNA and antibodies to HSV were detected more frequently in patients with BD than normal controls [5, 6]. *Streptococcus sanguis* was studied extensively as a candidate of the causative agent [7]. However, none of the pathogens has been proven to cause BD. Observations suggesting that several microbial agents were associated with the development of BD, rather, led to the hypothesis that common antigens such as heat shock protein (HSP) may be responsible for induction of the disease [8, 9].

HSP is highly immunogenic antigen and provokes prominent immune responses. HSP has highly conserved amino acid sequence throughout prokaryotic and eukaryotic kingdoms. Indeed, pathogenic role of anti-HSP immune responses has been suggested in various autoimmune diseases including rheumatoid arthritis. We here review the role of anti-HSP60 autoimmune responses in patients with BD.

ANTIGEN SPECIFIC RESPONSES
AGAINST HSP65 DERIVED PEPTIDES

There is ample evidence suggesting that HSP60/65 is involved in the pathogenesis of BD (Table 1). Lehner et al. first described increased IgA and IgG antibodies to HSP65 in sera from BD patients [7]. The anti-human HSP65 antibodies cross-reacted with streptococcal HSP60. They subsequently identified four peptides derived from the bacterial HSP60 and the corresponding peptides of human HSP65 that stimulated T cells specifically in patients with BD [10]. Similar result has been reproduced in Turkey [11]. B cell epitope mapping study supported importance of the four epitopes of HSP in patients with BD [12].

Table 1　Involvement of anti-HSP60/65 immune responses in BD.

---

1. Increased IgA and IgG antibodies to HSP65 in sera from BD patients [7].
2. Increased IgA and IgG antibodies to HSP65 in cerebrospinal fluid from BD patients having neurological manifestations [16].
3. Four bacterial HSP60-derived peptides and the corresponding human HSP65 peptides stimulated T cells from BD patients in UK and Turkey [10,11].
4. B cell epitopes overlapped with the four T cell epitopes in BD patients [12].
5. Peptide 336–351 is a dominant T cell epitope in Japanese BD patients [13].
6. Peptide 336–351 provokes uveitis in rat model of BD [14,15].

Noboru Suzuki et al.

Among the four peptides, we found that the peptide 336–351, Hu-18, provoked vigorous proliferation of T cells from BD patients in Japan, especially those with active uveitis [13]. The epitope was specific for BD, because no significant response was detected in patients with RA and normal controls. Interestingly, immunization with Hu-18 led to development of experimental uveitis in Lewis rats [14,15]. These data suggest that autoimmune responses to HSP are involved in the development of BD.

Increased expression of HSP65 antigens were shown in the epidermal cells and infiltrating mononuclear cells of skin lesions and circulating leukocytes from BD patients [9], suggesting that aberrant expression of HSP65 are, at least in part, responsible for induction of the HSP specific autoimmune responses in BD.

CHARACTERIZATION
OF PATHOGENIC T CELLS

We found that CD4+, but not CD8+ T cells responded to Hu-18 in BD patients [13]. Experimental uveitis is mediated by CD4+T cells, whereas CD8+ T cells suppresses the disease [15]. These findings indicate that CD4+ T cells play a pathologic role in the development of BD.

We studied T cell receptor (TCR) utilized by Hu-18 responding T cells in patients with BD [13]. Flowcytometric analysis revealed that T cells expressing particular V beta subfamily expanded selectively in response to Hu-18 stimulation *in vitro*. TCR Vbeta usage of the Hu-18 responding T cells was different from patient to patient. For example, when PBL were stimulated with Hu-18 for 7 days, Vbeta18.1 bearing cells increased from 1.6% to 50.3% in a patient. In another patient, Vbeta5a bearing cells increased from 4.1% to 40.1% in response to the same stimulation.

To further examine the T cell clonality, we analyzed the Vbeta specific RT-PCR products by using single strand conformational polymorphism (SSCP) technique, which can detect monoclonal accumulation of the T cells [13]. PBL stimulated with Hu-18 showed oligoclonal T cell accumulation, indicating that the peptide stimulated T cells in a conventional antigen-specific fashion. The oligoclonal expansion of Hu-18 specific T cells became evident in clinical exacerbations, while it disappeared during remission. The same T cell clones re-expanded in another clinical attack, suggesting the direct involvement of anti-Hu-18 specific T cell responses in the pathogenesis of BD.

CYTOKINE PRODUCTION

It is evident that proinflammatory cytokines are involved in the development of BD [9] (Table 2). Preferential Th1 cell activation is one of the most important abnormalities of cytokine network in BD. In our study, Hu-18 stimulated-PBL secreted significantly higher amounts of IL-12, TNF-alpha, and IFN-gamma in patients having active symptoms than those in remission and normal controls. Immunohistochemical studies revealed that infiltrating mononuclear cells synthesized IFN-gamma, but not IL-4, in

Table 2 Abnormalities of cytokine production in BD.

____

1. Plasma levels of proinflammatory cytokines are elevated; IL-1beta, IL-8, TNF-alpha [17–19].
2. IL-12 and IFN-gamma are increased in sera from active BD patients and CSF from those having neurological manifestations [9, 20].
3. IFN-gamma producing T cells are increased in circulation and are accumulated in skin lesions [9, 20] .
4. IL-4 suppresses HSP-induced experimental uveitis in rats [15].
____

skin lesions from BD patients. IL-4, IL-10, and TGF-beta were exclusively produced by Hu-18 stimulated PBL in patients during remission. In HSP60-induced experimental uveitis, exogenous IL-4 was shown to suppress the disease progression [15]. Thus, it is plausible that Th1 cytokines promote the disease, whereas Th2 cytokines play a protective role in BD.

It has been reported that excessive IL-12 secretion contributes to development and outgrowth of autoreactive Th1 cells in BD patients having active disease [20]. We recently found that IL-12 receptor (IL-12R) expressing T cells, which have a high IFN-gamma producing potential, were increased in PBL from BD patients with active disease. These data suggest that IL-12/IL-12R system plays a vital role in Th1 polarization during active disease in patients with BD. IL-12R expression on circulating T cells might be a simple marker to monitor the disease activity, as well as serum level of IL-12.

CYTOKINES AS THERAPEUTIC TARGETS IN BD

Cytokines are possible therapeutic targets in BD as have been in various autoimmune diseases. A simple approach is to neutralize pathogenic cytokines. A clinical trial of anti-TNF-alpha monoclonal antibody for serious uveitis is undergoing in Japan. The preliminary result looks promising. Thalidomide that inhibits actions of TNF is under consideration for clinical application in Japan [21].

Excessive Th1 cell activity has been detected in patients with BD and suppressive effect of IL-4 on the disease manifestation was shown in the rat model of BD [15]. Thus, correction of the Th1/Th2 imbalance is an alternative therapeutic approach.

We have previously characterized Txk, a member of Tec family tyrosine kinases in human T cells. Txk is selectively expressed on Th1 and Th0 cells, but not Th2 cells [22]. Upon stimulation, Txk translocates from cytoplasm to nuclei and selectively upregulates Th1 specific cytokine gene transcription, presumably as a Th1 cell specific transcription factor. In concordant with Th1 polarization in BD, immunoblotting and immunostaining studies revealed that circulating and infiltrating T cells from the patients expressed excessive Txk protein. We here propose that Txk is a novel therapeutic target in BD, because antisense oligonucleotide to Txk gene selectively inhibits Th1 cytokine production [22]. We are now investigating a pharmacological target in the Txk-mediated signaling pathway at a molecular level.

                                    Noboru Suzuki et al.

CONCLUSIONS

1. Autoreactive T cells against HSP60/65 play a pathogenic role in BD. The clonal size of the autoreactive T cells is closely correlated with the disease activity.
2. Th1 cytokines are involved in exacerbation of the disease, whereas Th2 cytokines play a protective role.
3. Correction of Th1/Th2 imbalance is a possible therapeutic target.

ACKNOWLEDGEMENT

Supported by a research grant from the Behçet's Disease Research Committee of Japan, the Ministry of Health and Welfare of Japan, and by a research grant from SRF Foundation, Tokyo, Japan.

REFERENCES

1. Sakane, T., Kotani, H., Takada, S., and Tsunematsu, T., *Arthritis Rheum.* 25: 1343–1351, 1982.
2. Sakane, T., Suzuki, N., Ueda, Y., Takada, S., Murakawa, Y., Hoshino, T., Niwa, Y., and Tsunematsu, T., *Arthritis Rheum.* 29:371–378, 1986.
3. Suzuki, N., Sakane, T., Ueda, Y., and Tsunematsu, T., *Arthritis Rheum.* 29: 212–219, 1986.
4. Rogers, R.S. 3rd., Sams, W.M. Jr., and Shorter, RG., *Arch. Dermatol.* 109: 361–363, 1974.
5. Hamza, M., Elleuch, M., Slim, A., Hamzaoui, K., and Ayed, K., *Clin. Rheumatol.* 9: 498–500, 1990.
6. Studd, M., McCance, D.J., and Lehner, T., *J. Med. Microbiol.* 34:39–43, 1991.
7. Lehner, T., Lavery, E., Smith, R., van der Zee, R., Mizushima, Y., and Shinnick, T., *Infect. Immun.* 59:1434–1441, 1991.
8. Sakane, T., Takeno, M., Suzuki, N., and Inaba, G., *N. Engl. J. Med.* 341:1284–1291, 1999.
9. Lehner, T., *Behçet's disease.* pp.3–18, Library of Congress Cataloging in Publication Data, 2001.
10. Pervin, K., Childerstone, A., Shinnick, T., Mizushima, Y., van der Zee, R., Hasan, A., and Vaughan, R, and Lehner, T., *J. Immunol.* 151:2273–2282, 1993.
11. Direskeneli, H., Eksioglu-Demiralp, E., Yavuz, S., Ergun, T., Shinnick, T., Lehner, T., and Akoglu, T., *J. Rheumatol.* 27:708–713, 2000.
12. Direskeneli, H., Hasan, A., Shinnick, T., Mizushima, Y., van der Zee, R., Fortune, F., Stanford, M.R., and Lehner, T., *Scand. J. Immunol.* 43:464–471, 1996.
13. Kaneko, S., Suzuki, N., Yamashita, N., Nagafuchi, H., Nakajima, T., Wakisaka, S., Yamamoto, S., and Sakane, T., *Clin. Exp. Immunol.* 108: 204–212, 1997.
14. Stanford, M.R., Kasp, E., Whiston, R., Hasan, A., Todryk, S., Shinnick, T., Mizushima, Y., Dumonde, D.C., van der Zee, R., and Lehner, T., *Clin. Exp. Immunol.* 97:226–231,1994.
15. Hu, W., Hasan, A., Wilson, A., Stanford, M.R., Li-Yang, Y., Todryk, S., Whiston, R., Shinnick, T., Mizushima, Y., van der Zee, R., and Lehner, T., *Eur. J. Immunol.* 28:2444–2455, 1998.
16. Tasci, B., Direskeneli, H., Serdaroglu, P., Akman-Demir, G., Eraksoy, M., and Saruhan-Direskeneli, G., *Clin. Exp. Immunol.* 113:100–104, 1998.
17. Yosipovitch, G., Shohat, B., Bshara, J., Wysenbeek, A., and Weinberger, A., *Isr. J. Med. Sci.* 31:345–348, 1995.

18. al-Dalaan, A., al-Sedairy, S., al-Balaa, S., al-Janadi, M., Elramahi, K., Bahabri, S., and Siddiqui, S., *J. Rheumatol.* 22:904–907, 1995.
19. Kosar, A., Haznedaroglu, S., Karaaslan, Y., Buyukasik, Y., Haznedaroglu, I.C., Ozath, D., Sayinalp, N., Ozcebe, O., Kirazli, S., and Dundar, S., *Rheumatol. Int.* 19:11–14, 1999.
20. Frassanito, M.A., Dammacco, R., Cafforio, P., and Dammacco, F., *Arthritis Rheum.* 42: 1967–1974, 1999.
21. Sakane, T., and Takeno, M., *Expert Opin. Investig. Drugs* 9:1993–2005, 2000.
22. Kashiwakura, J., Suzuki, N., Nagafuchi, H., Takeno, M., Takeba, Y., Shimoyama, Y., and Sakane, T., *J. Exp. Med.* 190:1147–1154, 1999.

Noboru Suzuki et al.

MINORU KIMURA, TAKAHIRO KIMURA, MASAHIRO SATO, TOSHITERU
WATANABE, SHIGEAKI OHNO, HIDETOSHI INOKO AND EI-ICHI NOMURA

10. An Attempt To Create A Behçet's Disease Model In Mice

ABSTRACT

To examine the pathogenesis of Behçet's disease (BD), we have generated transgenic
mice carrying the Major histocompatibility complex (MHC) class I related gene
A(*MICA*) or gene B(*MICB*) cDNA driven by cytomegalovirus enhancer and chicken
β-actin promoter (CAG promoter).

The *CAG-MICB* lines exhibited temporary skin lesions, as exemplified by hyperkeratosis, 50% increase in the number of white blood cells (WBCs) and reduction in
body weight comparing to their non-transgenic littermates. However, active lesions
mimicking BD were not observed in these mice. *CAG-MICA* mice exhibited altered
phenotypes such as reduction in the number of RBCs, alopecia and immune system
abnormalities, but never exhibited temporary skin lesions as observed in CAG-MICB
mice. We have also made *B51 x β2m* double transgenic mice through mating and these
mice exhibited enhanced expression of HLA-B51 molecules on the surface of lymphoid cells, but did not manifest any overt BD-associated phenotypic characteristics
throughout life.

KEYWORDS: Animal model; transgenic mice; *MICA* gene; *MICB* gene; *HLA-B51
gene;* β2 microglobulin

INTRODUCTION

Behçet's disease (BD) is characterized by four major signs and symptoms: oral apthous ulcers, skin lesions, ocular symptoms, and genital ulcerations, and occasionally
by inflammation in tissues and organs throughout the body. BD is thus considered a
refractory systemic inflammation disorder. It is well established that BD is associated
with the *HLA-B51* allele, which is relatively frequent, ranging from 45 to 60% in
incidence in many different ethnic groups including Asian and Eurasian populations

from Japan and the Middle East [1]. However, it is unclear whether *HLA-B51* itself or a closely linked gene is responsible for susceptibility to BD.

Recently, our group [2] found a triplet repeat microsatellite polymorphism of (GCT/AGC)n in the transmembrane (TM) region of the *MICA* gene [3]. *MICA* is a member of a novel family of the human major histocompatibility complex (MHC) class I genes termed *MIC* (MHC class I chain-related genes), and is located near the *HLA-B* gene on the short arm of human chromosome 6 [3]. Mizuki et al. [2] found 5 distinct alleles of (GCT/AGC)n in *MICA* using HLA homozygous B cell lines. Of 5 alleles tested one contained one additional base insertion that caused a framshift mutation resulting in a premature termination codon in the TM region. This particular allele was thought to encode a soluble, secreted form of the *MICA* molecule. Analysis of a total of 77 Japanese patients with BD, which is known to be associated with *HLA-B51*, revealed that the $(GCT/AGC)_6$ allele was strongly associated with BD in these patients [2]. These findings suggested that *MICA* is closely associated with BD rather than *HLA-B51*. Furthermore, our group [4] also reported the presence of allelic variants of the *MICB* gene [3], another member of *MIC* and which has a high degree of similarity to *MICA* as noted below, through screening of a total of 46 HLA homozygous B-cell lines. The number of *MICA* (more than 54 alleles) and *MICB* alleles (more than 16 alleles) has increased [4,5; S. Bahram, personal communication].

Of 5 *MIC* members (*MICB, MICA, MICC, MICD,* and *MICE* in order from centro- to telomere) so far identified in the *MIC* gene family, only the *MICA* and *MICB* genes are expressed [6]. The *MICA* and *MICB* genes are located respectively 46.4 kb and 141.2 kb centromeric to the *HLA-B* gene, with opposite transcriptional orientation [7]. The full-length *MICB* cDNA sequence is 2376 bp [8], compared with the 1382 bp *MICA* transcript, the difference in length due to a large 3' untranslated sequence in *MICB*. However, the lengths of *MICA* and *MICB* open reading frames (ORFs) are equal, and both transcripts encode a 383 amino acid polypeptide chain with molecular weight of 43 kDa with 83% identity at the amino acid level [3,8]. In contrast to typical *MHC* class I genes, both *MICA* and *MICB* transcripts are absent from cells of lympho-hematopoeitic cell lines such as T cells, B cells and monocytes, but are strongly transcribed in fibroblasts and epithelial cell lines [3,8]. Expression levels of both *MICA* and *MICB* transcripts are not affected by type I and II interferons [3], which are known to markedly upregulate the level of typical *MHC* class I gene expression, but are responsive to cell-stress due to heat shock responsive element in their promoters [6,9]. *MICA* and *MICB* are conserved in most if not all mammals but appear to be missing in the mouse [3,8]. Unlike all other MHC class I and related molecules, both *MICA* and *MICB* molecules were not associated with β_2-microglobulin (β2m) and cytosolic peptides. Interestingly, recent work has demonstrated cell-surface expression of the highly glycosylated *MICA* molecule exclusively in the gastrointestinal epithelium [9]. Although the amino acid sequence of both *MICA* and *MICB* molecules is to some extent similar to those of HLA class I antigen molecules (approximately 30%), analysis of the predicted 3D structure revealed that both *MICA* and *MICB* molecules resemble the mouse nonclassical MHC class I T10[b] and T22[b], which are recognized by $\gamma\delta$ T cells [3]. *MICA* is also recognized by NK cells. Therefore, *MICA* and the closely related *MICB* might act as a ligand for a subset of T cells in the intestinal intraepithelial lymphocyte compartment [9]. Given the unusual characteristics of the *MICA* and *MICB* genes and the evidence of the diverse functions of class I-related molecules in antigen presentation and T cell recognition, it appears that *MICA* and *MICB* are probably unrelated to conventional MHC class I antigen presentation and may serve a specialized T cell immune surveillance function.

T lymphocytes are generally thought to play roles in the pathogenesis and/or modification of the clinical course of BD, since i) there is functional aberration of a suppressor T cell subset derived from patients with pre-active BD [10], and ii) γδ T cells are the major cell type among infiltrating lymphocytes and their numbers are increased in the peripheral blood of BD patients [11,12]. Based on this background, we postulated that *MICA* and *MICB* moleucles are epitopes recognized by γδ T cells, and that once γδ T cells are activated after expression of *MICA* and *MICB*, they elicit BD-associated phenotypes. In this study, we introduced a human *MICA* or *MICB* cDNA-expressing unit (transgene) into the mouse genome using transgenesis technique [13] to obtain information on the functions of *MICA* and *MICB*, and on the possible involvement of these genes in the pathogenesis of BD.

RESULTS

cDNAs coding for *MICA* (carrying 5 repetitive alanines in the TM region and corresponding to the normal allele) [3] and *MICB* [8] were kindly provided from Dr. Bahram. Each cDNA was ligated to a CAG promoter system consisting of cytomgalovirus enhancer and promoter and the 1st intron of the chicken β-actin gene [14], which confers strong and ubiquitous expression of the downstream cDNA sequence in mice [15,16]. The resulting constructs for transgenic mouse production are shown in Figure 1. Production of transgenic mice by pronuclear injection of transgene was performed as described previously [17].

Of more than 30 F0 mice for each transgene obtained, six and ten mice were identified to be transgenic by PCR analysis of genomic DNA from biopsied tails.

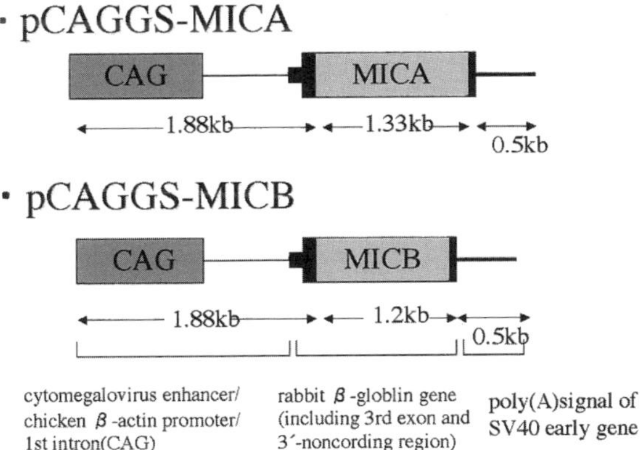

Figure 1 The *CAG-MICA* and *CAG-MICB* transgene constructs. Each fragment containing *MICA* or *MICB* cDNA was inserted into the *Eco* RI site present in the 3rd exon of rabbit β-globin gene in pCAGGS vector [14].

Some F0 mice were unable to transmit their transgenes to F1 offspring, probably due to mosaicism for the transgene. When F1 or F2 offspring of the established lines were examined for transgene expression at Northern level, expression of *MICA* and *MICB* mRNA appeared to be low (data not shown). We thus failed to obtain a high-expression transgenic line for each cDNA. Expression of *MICA* and *MICB* molecules thus appears be somewhat toxic to mice.

When F1 offspring of 3 independent *CAG-MICB* lines that had been proven to be expressed by RT-PCR analyses were examined for blood components, they all exhibited 50% increase in the number of white blood cells (WBCs) compared to their non-transgenic littermates (Fig. 2). These *CAG-MICB* lines also exhibited 60–70% reduction in body weight compared to their non-transgenic littermates at 3 to 4 months after birth (Fig. 3).

The most striking feature of these *CAG-MICB* lines was temporary skin lesions with exfoliation or scaling (Fig. 4). This phenotype first appeared around 10 days after birth and disappeared after 2 weeks of age. It was repeatedly observed in the transgenic offspring (heterozygous for the transgene) of 3 independent *CAG-MICB* lines examined.

Histopathological analyses of the skin of young mice exhibiting skin abnormalities revealed hyperkeratosis of epidermis and thickening of the granular layer (Fig. 5). Slight infiltration of inflammatory cells was also observed in the dermis. No perivascular infiltration typically found in psoriasis vulgaris was observed. This abnormal phenotype thus resembles human ichthyosis. Other main abnormalities associated with BD (such as oral apthous ulcers, ocular symptoms and genital ulcerations) were not observed in the *CAG-MICB* lines.

In the *CAG-MICA* transgenic mice, at least three phenotypic alterations including reduction in the number of red blood cells (RBCs), alopecia and increased production of serum IgG were observed. The average number of RBCs in the non-transgenic control mice was approximately 10×10^6 per μl, while that in the *CAG-MICA* transgenic lines was approximately 7×10^6 per μl (Fig. 6). Of a total of 3 *CAG-MICA* lines examined, one line exhibited alopecia which commenced 2–3 weeks after birth (Fig. 7). Since alopecia is thought to be frequently associated with immune system abnomalities, we next examined the amount of serum IgG by Ouchterlony's test. The results are summarized in Figure 8. Although the difference between the *CAG-MICA* transgenic lines and non-transgenic control appears to be small, it was significant ($P<0.05$).

Besides *MICA* and *MICB*, the *HLA-B51* allele is thought to be one of the genes principally responsible for the pathogenesis of BD [1]. In a previous study using transgenic mice expressing human *HLA-B51* molecule, phenotypic abnormalities associated with BD were not found in natural condition, but hyperfunction of neutrophils, which results in prodcution of substantial amounts of superoxide and is known to be closely associated with BD, was induced in the *HLA-B51* transgenic mice by administration of FMLP [18]. In the *HLA-B51* transgenic mice, the *HLA-B51* molecule might not have been fully expressed on the surface of lymphocytes, since human *HLA-B51* appears not to interact efficiently with the endogenous mouse *β2m* molecule. This may be supported by the following experiments. Transgenic rats expressing both human *HLA-B27* and human *β2m* genes developed a spontaneous in-

Minoru Kimura et al.

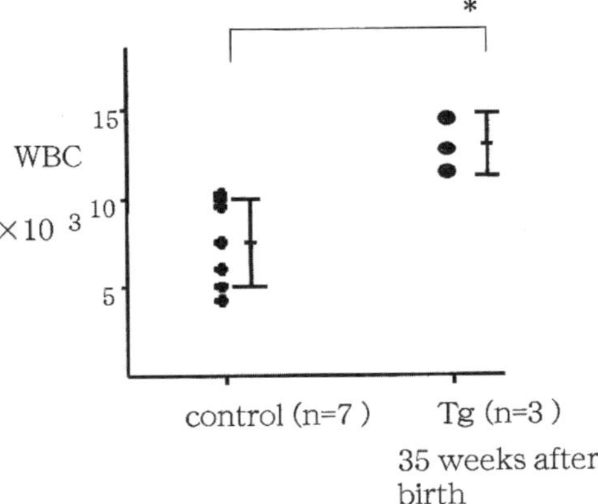

Figure 2 Comparison of the number of white blood cells (WBCs) between F1 transgenic (Tg) and non-transgenic (control) littermates of a *CAG-MICB* transgenic line. Blood was isolated from the tail and examined for number of WBCs using an automatic blood analyzer. The transgenic samples examined exhibited an approximately 50% increase in the number of WBCs compared with the non-transgenic samples.

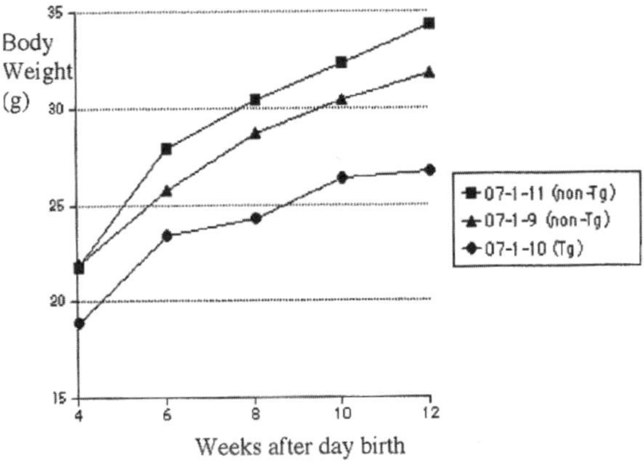

Figure 3 Comparison of the growth curves for F1 transgenic (Tg) and non-transgenic (non-Tg) littermates of a CAG-MICB transgenic line. The transgenic mice exhibited 30–40% reduction in body weight compared to their non-transgenic littermates throughout life.

flammatory disease [19], and transgenic mice expressing *HLA-B27* gene did not exhibit arthritis, either spontaneous or induced [20]. These findings suggest that the human *HLA-B27* molecule interacts more efficiently with human *β2m* than with mouse *β2m* , and that its expression is hampered by the presence of mouse *β2m*. This hypothesis was confirmed by the observation that when *HLA-B27* transgene was introduced into *β2m*-deficient mice, spontaneous arthritis was observed in *HLA-B27* transgenic mice lacking murine *β2m* gene (B27+ β2m−/−) compared with *HLA-B27*

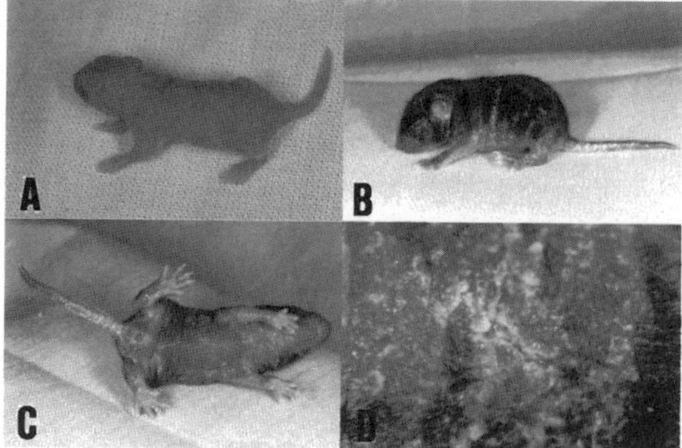

Figure 4 Skin lesion temporarily present in the *CAG-MICB* lines. A. A newborn transgenic mouse, aged 4 days, never exhibited any skin abnormality. B,C. The same pup shown in A, aged 8 days, began to exhibit clear skin lesions on both dorsal (B) and ventral (C) sides. D. The pup shown in B and C exhibited numerous scales on its skin surface.

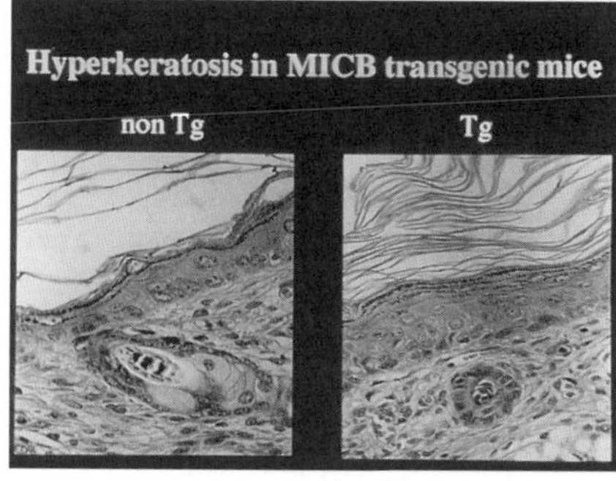

Figure 5 Hyperkeratosis of epidermis in the F1 offspring of a *CAG-MICB* line, aged 2 weeks. The transgenic (Tg) sample exhibited hyperkeratosis in its epidermis and thickening of the granular layer, while the non-transgenic (non Tg) sample did not.

transgenic mice carrying endogenous murine *β2m* gene (B27$^+$ β2m$^{+/-}$) [21]. In analogy with *HLA-B27*, we suspect that introduction of *HLA-B51* allele into mice expressing human *β2m* enhances expression of *HLA-B51* on the surface of lymphocytes, which may in turn increase the severity of BD-associated characteristics.

We produced double transgenic mice (hereafter termed *B51 x β2m*) by mating the *HLA-B51* transgenic mice ([18]; obtained from Dr. Takiguchi at Kumamoto University) with mice overexpressing human *β2m* (unpublished; obtained from Dr. Maruyama of Niigata University). Peripheral lymphocytes were collected from the *B51 x β2m* mice and non-transgenic mice, and examined for expression of MHC class I molecules with flow cytometric assay using anti-pan class I antibodies. The results are

Minoru Kimura et al.

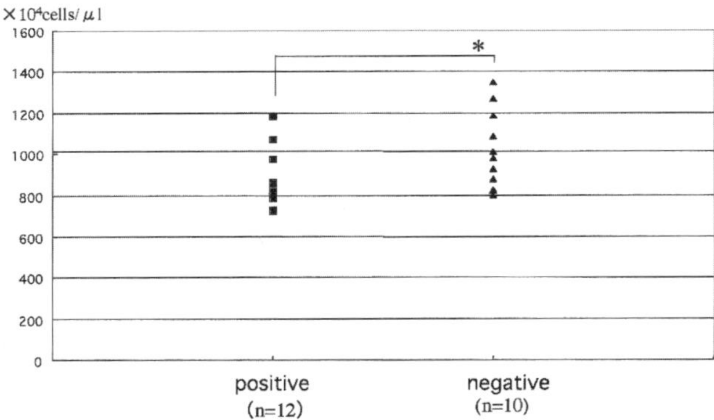

Figure 6 Comparison of the number of red blood cells (RBCs) in F1 offspring between transgenic (positive) and non-transgenic (negative) littermates of a *CAG-MICA* line. Blood was isolated from the tail of each mouse and examined for number of RBCs using an automated blood analyzer. The average number of RBCs in the *CAG-MICA* transgenic mice was approximately 7×10^6 /μl, while that in the non-transgenic mice was approximately 10×10^6 /μl.

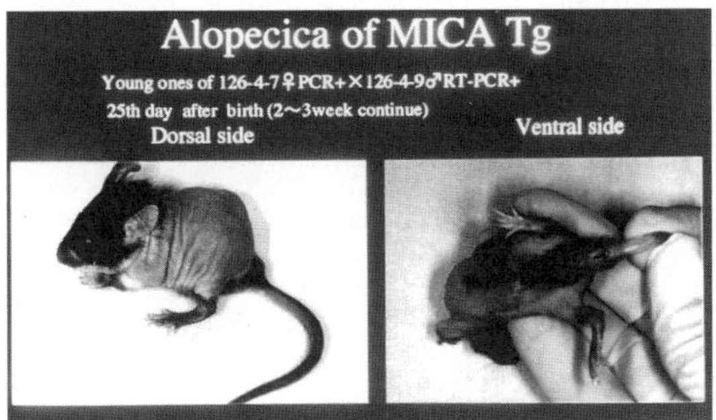

Figure 7 Alopecia found in one line of *CAG-MICA* transgenic mice.

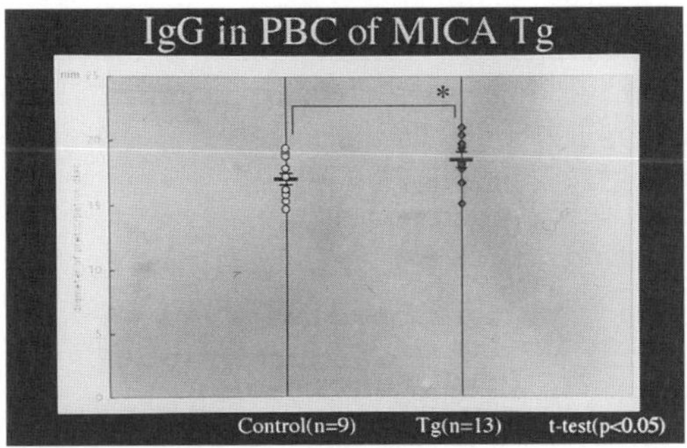

Figure 8 Comparison of the amount of serum IgG in F1 offspring between the transgenic (Tg) and non-transgenic (control) littermates of a *CAG-MICA* transgenic line, as evaluated by Ouchterlony's test. The transgenic samples exhibited a significant increase (p<0.05) in the amount of serum IgG compared with the non-transgenic samples. The longitudinal axis indicates the diameter (mm) of precipitation discs.

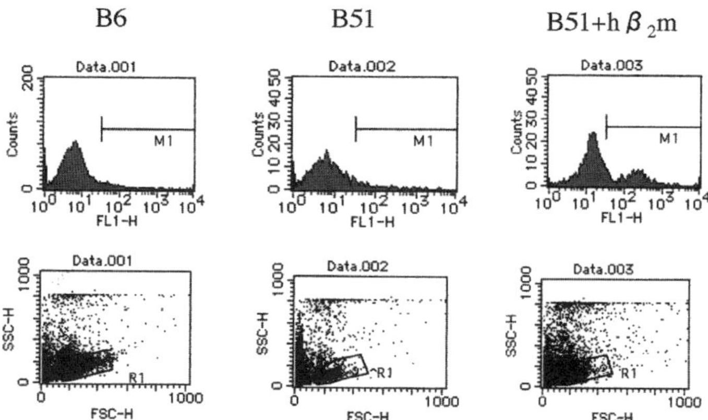

Figure 9 Cell-surface expression of human HLA-B51 molecules in lymphocytes of the B51 x β2m double transgenic mice. Peripheral lymphocytes were isolated from non-transgenic (B6), HLA-B51 transgenic (B51) and B51 x β2m double transgenic mice (B51 + hβ2m), and analyzed by flow cytometric assay using anti-pan class I antibodies, which can recognize both human HLA and murine H2 molecules. In each figure, a large peak on the left side indicates expression of endogenous murine H2 antigen on the cell-surface of lymphocytes. Notably, there is another prominant peak with a high degree of fluorescence in the B51 x β2m sample. This profile appears to correspond to the lymphocytes expressing human HLB-51 molecules on their cell-surface. In the HLA-B51 transgenic sample, a slight shoulder is observed on the right side of the control peak (corresponding to the murine H2-expressing lymphocytes) and appears to correspond to the human HLA-B51-expressing lymphocytes.

shown in Figure 9. These profiles indicated that human *HLA-B51* gene product was expressed more efficiently on the cell surface of lymphocytes of the *B51 x β2m* mice than that of the *HLA-B51* mice. However, no abnormalities such as ocular lesions mimicking BD were evident in any of these *B51 x β2m* mice yet examined. Experiments are in progress, particularly concerning possible abnormalities in the immune system in these *B51 x β2m* mice similar to those in *CAG-MICA* mice. Furthermore, we are planning to introduce *HLA-B51* x human *β2m* double transgenes into the mice lacking murine *β2m* gene (β2m$^{-/-}$). It is expected that mice (HLA-B51^{+} human β2m^{+} β2m$^{-/-}$) will express *HLA-B51* molecules more efficiently than the *B51 x β2m* mice in the absence of intrinsic H2 molecules.

CONCLUSION

Table 1 shows a summary of this study. *CAG-MICB* transgenic mice exhibited temporary skin lesions, as exemplified by hyperkeratosis, increase in the number of WBCs and reduction in body weight. However, active lesions mimicking BD were not observed in these mice. *CAG-MICB* mice appear to be an animal model of skin disease such as ichthyosis. *CAG-MICA* mice exhibited altered phenotypes such as reduction in the number of RBCs, alopecia and immune system abnormalities, but never exhib-

                                   Minoru Kimura et al.

Table 1 Summary of this study using transgenic mice.

Phenotypic alteration	Transgenic mice			
	CAG-MICA	*CAG-MICB*	*HLA-B51*	*B51 x β2m*
WBC	Unchanged	Increased	ND	ND
RBC	Decreased	Unchanged	ND	ND
Body weight	Unchanged	Decreased	Unchanged	Unchanged
IgG, IgA[a]	Increased	ND	ND	ND
Skin	alopecia	hyperkeratosis	Unchanged	Unchanged
Superoxide in neutrophils	ND	ND	Increased[b]	ND

[a]Determined by Ouchterlony's test.
[b]Only after induction with FMLP; cited from Takeno et al. (1995) Arthritis Rheumat 38, 426–433.

Abbreviations are: ND, not determined; RBC, red blood cell; WBC, white blood cell.

ited temporary skin lesions as observed in *CAG-MICB* mice. It remains unclear why the phenotypic abnormalities of the *CAG-MICA* and *CAG-MICB* mice differed, since *MICA* exhibits a high degree of similarity (83% homology at the amino acid level) to *MICB*. The TM region of *MICA* is known to be quite different (18 of 65 amino acid substitutions are clustered within this segment of 24 amino acids [6]) from that of *MICB*. This low degree of similarity in the TM region may cause the difference in phenotypes of *CAG-MICB* and *CAG-MICA* mice. Finally, *B51 x β2m* double transgenic mice exhibited immune system abnormalities, but did not manifest any overt BD-associated phenotypic characteristics throughout life.

In this study, we attempted to produce a BD model by expressing *MICB, MICA* or both *HLA-B51* and *β2m* in mice, but failed, although immune system abnormalities and temporary skin lesions were elicited in these mice. The following studies are now in progress to create a BD mouse model: i) introduction of *MICB, MICA* or *HLA-B51* gene or these three genes into mice ($β2m^{-/-}$) lacking the *β2m* gene through mating, and ii) introduction of the entire BD-susceptible region spanning 10–50 kb isolated from BD patients into the mouse genome by the transgenesis method.

ACKNOWLEDGEMENTS

This work was supported by the grants of the Ministry of Education, Science, Sports and Culture, Japan and the Ministry of Health and Welfare, Japan.

REFERENCES

1. Ohno, S., Ohguchi, M., Hirose, S., Matsudam H., Wakisaka, A. and Aizawa, M., *Arch. Ophthalmol.* 100: 1455–1458, 1982.
2. Mizuki, N., Ota. M., Kimura, M., Ohno, S., Ando, H., Katsuyama, Y., Yamazaki, Y., Watanabe, K., Goto, K., Nakamura, S. Bahram, S. and Inoko, H., *Proc. Natl. Acad. Sci. USA* 94: 1298–1303, 1997.

3. Bahram, S., Bresnahan, M., Geraghty, D.E. and Spies, T., *Proc. Natl. Acad. Sci. USA* 91: 6259–6263, 1994.

4. Ando, H., Mizuki, N., Ota, M., Yamazaki, M., Ohno, S., Goto, K., Miyata, Y., Wakisaka, K., Bahram, S. and Inoko, H., *Immunogenetics* 46: 499–508, 1997.

5. Fodil, N., Laloux, L., Wanner, V., Pellet, P., Hauptmann, G., Mizuki, N., Inoko, H., Spies, T., Theodorou, I. and Bahram, S., *Immunogenetics* 44: 351–357, 1996.

6. Bahram, S. and Spies, T., *Res. Immunol.* 147: 328–333, 1996.

7. Mizuki, N., Ando, H., Kimura, M., Ohno, S., Miyata, S., Yamazaki, M., Tashiro, H., Watanabe, K., Ono, A., Taguchi, S., Sugawara, C., Fukuzumi, Y., Okumura, K., Goto, K., Ishihara, M., Nakamura, S., Yonemoto, J., Kikuti, Y-Y., Shiina, T., Chen, L., Ando, A., Ikemura, T. and Inoko, H., *Genomics* 42: 55–66, 1997.

8. Bahram, S. and Spies, T., *Immunogenetics* 43: 230–233, 1996.

9. Groh, V., Bahram, S., Bauer, S., Herman, A., Beauchamp, M. and Spies, T., *Proc. Natl. Acad. Sci. USA* 93: 12445–12450, 1996.

10. Sakane, T., Kotani, H., Takada, S. and Tsunematsu, T., *Arthritis Rheum.* 25: 1343–1351, 1982.

11. Fortune, F., Walker, J. and Lehner, T., *Clin. Exp. Immunol.* 82: 326–332, 1990.

12. Suzuki, Y., Hoshi, K., Matsuda, T. and Mizushima, Y., *J. Rheumatol.* 19: 588–592, 1992.

13. Gordon, J.W., Scangos, G.A., Plotkin, D.J., Barbosa, J.A. and Ruddle, F.H., *Proc. Natl. Acad. Sci. USA* 77: 7380–7384, 1980.

14. Niwa, H., Yamamura, K. and Miyazaki, J., *Gene* 108: 193–200, 1991.

15. Ishii, M., Tashiro, F., Hagiwara, S., Toyonaga, T., Hashimoto, C., Takei, I., Yamamura, K. and Miyazaki, J., *Endocr. J.* 41(Suppl.): S9-S16, 1994.

16. Sato, M., Kawarabayashi, T., Shoji, M., Kobayashi, T., Hirai, S. and Tada, N., *Transgenics* 2: 153–159, 1997.

17. Hogan, B., Costantini, F. and Lacy, E., *Manipulating the Mouse Embryo: A Laboratory Manual*, Cold Spring Harbor Laboratory, Cold Spring Harbor, NY, 1986.

18. Takeno, M., Kariyone, A., Yamashita, N., Takiguchi, M., Mizushuma, Y., Kaneoka, H. and Sakane, T., *Arthritis Rheum.* 38: 426–433, 1995.

19. Hammer, R.E., Maika, S.D., Richardson, J.A., Tang, J.-P. and Taurog, J.D., *Cell* 63: 1099–1112, 1990.

20. Nickerson, C.L., Hanson, J. and David, C.S., *J. Exp. Med.* 172: 1255–1261, 1990.

21. Khare, S.D., Luthra, H.S. and David, C.S., *J. Exp. Med.* 182: 1153–1158, 1995.

Minoru Kimura et al.

MITSUHIRO TAKENO, YOSHIHIRO SHIMOYAMA, HIROKO NAGAFUCHI,
NOBORU SUZUKI AND TSUYOSHI SAKANE

11. Neutrophil Hyperfunction in Behçet's Disease

ABSTRACT

Neutrophil hyperfunction is a hallmark of pathological features in Behçet's disease. We found that HLA-B51, which is the most well defined genetic marker in the disease, is responsible for the neutrophil abnormality at least in part. As shown in human study, neutrophils expressing HLA-B51 molecules in the transgenic mice revealed an increased H_2O_2 production in response to formyl methonine-leucine-phenylalanin when compared with controls. However, neutrophil hyperactivity in HLA-B51 transgenic mice was not sufficient for development of clinical manifestations, suggesting that additional genetic or environmental factors are also necessary for development of the disease.

We found that circulating neutrophils in patients with Behçet's disease spontaneously produce inflammatory cytokines. Especially in patients having active disease, neutrophils synthesize IL-12 and IL-18, which stimulate Th1 cells. Thus, neutrophils are implicated in the preferential activation of Th1 immune responses during active disease. These data support the idea that neutrophil is a therapeutic target in Behçet's disease.

KEYWORDS: neutrophil; HLA-B51; Th1; NF-kB

INTRODUCTION

Neutrophil hyperfunction is one of the characteristic features in Behçet's disease (BD) [1]. BD neutrophils show various functional and phenotypical abnormalities, which are involved in the pathophysiology of the disease; an increased chemotactic activity and upregulated adhesion molecules contribute to abnormal neutrophil accumulation in the lesions and excessive superoxides and proteolytic enzymes secreted by neutrophils are responsible for tissue injuries. Neutrophil is one of therapeutic targets in BD, as colchicine, which has inhibitory effects on neutrophil chemotaxis and neutrophil-endothelial cell interaction through adhesion molecules, has been introduced into the first line of therapies for BD in Japan [2].

Nevertheless, it is uncertain what causes neutrophil hyperfunction in BD. In spite of a close association of HLA-B51 with BD, the pathogenic role remains undetermined. We here review the implication of HLA-B51 in neutrophil hyperfunction on the basis of studies in human and HLA-B51 transgenic (Tg) mice [3–5].

We also focus cytokine production by neutrophils in patients with BD. Neutrophils had been recognized as exclusive terminal effector cells in inflammatory sites until recent studies revealed that neutrophils produce various cytokines, which regulate the immune system including Th1 versus Th2 balance. We show the possible role of neutrophil-derived cytokines in the development of BD.

NEUTROPHIL HYPERFUNCTION IN HLA-B51 TARNSGENIC MICE

We and others have demonstrated that HLA-B51 is implicated in neutrophil hyperfunction as shown in Table 1 [3–5]. However, it is difficult to determine whether the HLA-B51 antigen itself is primarily responsible for the neutrophil hyperfunction.

To this end, we generated HLA-B51 Tg mice as described elsewhere [5]. The transgene was derived from a healthy donor having HLA-B*5101, which is the most frequent subtype of HLA-B51 in both healthy controls and BD patients. We found that neutrophils from HLA-B51 transgenic mice produced significantly higher amounts of H_2O_2 in response to formyl methonine-leucine-phenylalanin (fMLP) than those from wild type and HLA-B35 Tg mice [5]. On the other hand, no difference was seen in PMA- or opsonized zymosan-induced H_2O_2 production among three groups. While fMLP triggers respiratory burst by primed neutrophils, PMA or opsonized zymosan can stimulate unprimed neutrophils to produce superoxide. The data suggest that neutrophils are primed *in vivo* and ready to respond to fMLP in HLA-B51 Tg mice, whereas those are resting in control mice. It is likely that the HLA-B51 antigen itself is directly involved in the neutrophil hyperactivity, though the precise mechanism is unknown.

It has been controversial whether the susceptibility to BD is determined by the HLA-B51 or nearby other gene in linkage disequilibrium with HLA-B51. Extensive genetic studies have not identified any genes that have a stronger association with BD than the HLA-B51 gene. The facts also support that the HLA-B51 antigen may be primarily involved in the disease.

Nonetheless, we did not find any clinical and pathological findings resembling human BD in the HLA-B51 Tg mice (Table 2). Rather, it is plausible that other genetic or environmental factors are also implicated in development of BD.

Table 1   Implications of HLA-B51 in human neutrophil function.

1. Enhanced neutrophil chemotaxis is associated with HLA-B51 positive BD patients, but not negative patients [3].
2. Neutrophils from HLA-B51 positive healthy individuals show an increased chemotaxis and superoxide production when compared with HLA-B51 negative healthy individuals [4].
3. Neutrophils from HLA-B51 positive individuals synthesize higher amounts of superoxide in response to fMLP than those from negative individuals [5].

Mitsuhiro Takeno et al.

Table 2 Features of HLA-B51 Tg mice.

| | superoxide production | | histological findings | clinical manifestations |
	fMLP-induced	PMA-induced		
HLA-B51 Tg	+	++	-	-
HLA-B35 Tg	-	++	-	-
Wild type	-	++	-	-

SPONTANEOUS CYTOKINE PRODUCTION BY NEUTROPHILS

Neutrophils reveal various functional abnormalities as effecter cells in patients with BD. We here focused on cytokine production by neutrophils. RT-PCR techniques revealed that neutrophils from healthy donors did not express mRNA of IL-1alpha, IL-18 and TNF-alpha at all, whereas they did express mRNA of these cytokines in response to lipopolysaccharide *in vitro*. In contrast, freshly isolated neutrophils from BD patients expressed mRNA of TNF-alpha and IL-1alpha, irrespective of their disease activity. IL-18 mRNA was also detected in neutrophils from patients having active disease but not those in remission.

We measured IL-12 in the neutrophil culture supernatants by ELISA, because it is hard to assess the synthesis of bioactive IL-12p70 heterodimer by using the RT-PCR technique. We found that neutrophils spontaneously secreted substantial amounts of IL-12p70 in BD patients having active disease but not those with inactive disease and normal controls. However, there was no significant difference in IL-8 production by neutrophils between controls and BD patients, even those having active symptoms.

As summarized in Table 3, neutrophils spontaneously produce IL-1alpha and TNF-alpha in BD patients, irrespective of their disease activity. It is plausible that BD neutrophils are functionally upregulated not only as terminal effecter cells but also as afferent cells.

Proinflammatory cytokines have stimulatory effects on neutrophils. Elevated circulating levels of IL-1 and TNF-alpha, both of which are responsible for neutrophil priming, were noted in BD patients [6,7]. Our data suggest that neutrophil is one of the sources of these cytokines and that neutrophil-derived cytokines may activate neutrophils themselves in an autocrine fashion. On the other hand, our data did not support that neutrophils are major sources of IL-8, though the cytokine was also shown to be responsible for neutrophil activation and tissue infiltration in BD [8].

There is a striking difference in intracellular biochemical events between effector functions and cytokine production. Cytokine synthesis requires the gene activation

Table 3 Cytokine production by peripheral neutrophils and disease activity in BD patients.

	IL-1alfa	TNF-alfa	IL-12	IL-18	IL-8
healthy control	-	-	-	-	+
BD inactive	+	+	-	-	+
BD active	+	+	+	+	+

that is regulated by transcription factors, whereas superoxide production and chemotaxis do not. We examined activation of NF-kB, which is involved in gene transcription of TNF-alpha and IL-1alpha, in peripheral neutrophils from patients with BD. The gel shift assay demonstrated that NF-kB translocated from cytoplasm to nuclei in response to TNF-alpha or LPS in neutrophils from normal donors. In contrast, NF-kB is detected in nuclei of freshly isolated neutrophils from BD patients. The results suggest that the constitute activation of NF-kB in neutrophils leads to spontaneous production of IL-1alpha and TNF-alpha.

Our study also showed that the production of IL-12 and IL-18 is associated with clinical exacerbations. Both of the cytokines stimulate T cells to produce interferon (IFN)-gamma. To determine whether the neutrophil-derived cytokines affect T cell function, we measured IFN-gamma production by anti-CD3 monoclonal antibody (mAb)-stimulated T cells in presence of neutrophil supernatants. Indeed, a potent IFN-gamma inducing activity was detected in neutrophil supernatants from BD patients with active disease but not those in remission and normal controls. The findings were concordant with the cytokine profiles of neutrophils, suggesting that neutrophil-derived cytokines may contribute to the skewed Th1 cytokine production during the disease exacerbations [9,10].

CONCLUSIONS

1. The HLA-B51 antigen itself may be directly involved in the neutrophil hyperactivity, though the precise mechanism is unknown.
2. The HLA-B51 mice did not express clinicopathological findings like human BD, indicating that other genetic or environmental factors are also implicated in development of the disease.
3. Neutrophils spontaneously produce various cytokines, which may be implicated in the neutrophil activation, endothelial abnormalities and the Th1 shift in BD.

ACKNOWLEDGEMENT

Supported by a research grant from the Behçet's Disease Research Committee of Japan, the Ministry of Health and Welfare of Japan, and by a research grant from SRF Foundation, Tokyo, Japan.

REFERENCES

1. Sakane, T., Takeno, M., Suzuki, N., and Inaba, G., *N. Engl. J. Med.* 341:1284–1291, 1999.
2. Misushima, Y., Matsumura, N., Mori, N., Shimizu, T., Fukushima, B., Mimura, Y., Saito, K., and Sugiura, S., *Lancet* ii(8046):1037, 1977.
3. Chajek-Shaul, T. Pisanty, S., Knobler, H., Matzner, Y., Glick, M., Ron, N., Rosenman, E., Brautbar, C., *Am. J. Med.* 83:666–672, 1987.
4. Sensi, A., Gavioli, R., Spisani, S., Balboni, A., Melchiorri, L., Menicucci, A., Palumbo, G., Traniello, S., and Baricordi, O.R., *Dis. Markers* 9:327–331, 1991.

5. Takeno, M., Kariyone, A., Yamashita, N., Takiguchi, M., Mizushima, Y., Kaneoka, H., and Sakane, T., *Arthritis Rheum.* 38:426–433, 1995.

6. Yosipovitch, G., Shohat, B., and Bshara, J., J, Wysenbeek A, and Weinberger A., *Isr. J. Med. Sci.* 31:345–348, 1995.

7. Sayinalp, N., Ozcebe, O.I., Ozdemir, O., Haznedaroglu, I.C., Dundar, S., Kirazli, S., *J. Rheumatol.* 23:321–322, 1996

8. Katsantonis, J., Adler, Y., Orfanos, C.E., and Zouboulis, C.C., *Dermatol.* 201: 31–39, 2000

9. Kaneko, S., Suzuki, N., Yamashita, N., Nagafuchi, H., Nakajima, T., Wakisaka, S., Yamamoto, S., and Sakane, T., *Clin. Exp. Immunol.* 108:204–218, 1997.

10. Frassanito, M.A., Dammacco, R., Cafforio, P., and Dammacco, F., *Arthritis Rheum.* 42: 1967–1974, 1999

SEONGHYANG SOHN, EUN-SO LEE, DONGSINK BANG AND SUNGNACK LEE

12. Role of Infectious Organisms in Behçet's Disease

ABSTRACT

Etiopathological factors for Behçet's disease (BD) have been studied in various aspects. The streams have been connected to genetic background, infection, and autoimmune mechanism. The infectious etiopathology has been focused on the streptococcus and herpes simplex virus. Streptococcal components were deposited at the site of vessel wall and inflammatory infiltrates. Acquisition of hypersensitivity to streptococcal antigens may play an important role in the appearance of lesions in patients with BD. Viral etiology was first described and speculated by Hulusi Behçet in 1937. By the development of molecular biological tool, herpes simplex virus (HSV) etiology has taken an important part. Mouse model induced by HSV was very similar to the human patients in the appearance of symptoms, expression pattern of cytokines and efficiency of treatment. Human heat shock protein 60 kD has homology to mycobacterium HSP 65 kD, inducible by heat, stress and microorganism infection, could induce uveitis, one of major symptoms of this disease, in rat.

KEYWORDS: Herpes simplex virus; streptococcus; heat shock protein

Kaneko F et al. has suggested that infection induced allergy could react as an etiopathology of Behçet's disease (BD) (Table 1) [1,2]. They have also reported that streptococcal bacteria induced intense delayed hypersensitivity in BD patients compared to normal healthy controls in intradermal reaction. They tried to detect deposits of immune complexes in the aphthous ulcers and erythema nodosum (EN)-like eruptions. Deposits of IgM and positive fluorescence of anti-streptococcal serum were found in vessel walls and sites infiltrated by inflammatory cells [3]. In 1991, to elucidate the mechanism of the interaction between lymphocytes and neutrophils in the infiltrates of the BD lesions, Kaneko F et al. studied hypersensitivity against *S. salivarius*. They demonstrated that aphthous ulceration of patients with BD showed inflammatory infiltrates consisting of neutrophils and lymphocytes under the ulcer lesion. From the immunohistochemical results, deposits of streptococcal components were found at the site of inflammatory infiltrates. This finding suggested that streptococci in the oral

Table 1 Intradermal reaction in patients with Behçet's disease (n=84) and normal healthy controls (n=10).

Bacterial vaccines	Behçet's disease		Normal controls	
$(1\text{x}10^5 \text{ org/mL})$	15 min	48 h	15 min	48 h
S. pyogenes	7 ± 8	41 ± 15	11 ± 11	8 ± 6
S. viridans	8 ± 7	46 ± 11	4 ± 4	2 ± 3
S. non-hemolyticus	7 ± 7	35 ± 14	5 ± 5	3 ± 4
S. faecalis	10 ± 8	10 ± 19	12 ± 11	0
Pneumococcus	16 ± 10	32 ± 14	8 ± 9	3 ± 4
E. coli	6 ± 7	16 ± 11	2 ± 1	1 ± 2
H. influenzae	11 ± 10	15 ± 15	9 ± 13	11 ± 12
Sta. aureus	8 ± 7	12 ± 13	3 ± 7	0 ± 1
Sta. epidermidis	5 ± 7	6 ± 7	2 ± 7	1 ± 2
Prot. vulgaris	10 ± 16	28 ± 13	6 ± 6	17 ± 4
Pseud. aeruginosa	1 ± 1	22 ± 11	2 ± 3	5 ± 0
SK-SD (50 U/mL)		9 ± 12		20 ± 9
Saline		2 ± 4		0 ± 1

The numbers denote mean SD of (Length+Width)/2 of erythemas

cavity played an important role in aphthous ulcer formation [4]. From these results, Kaneko et al. concluded that the acquisition of hypersensitivity to streptococcal antigens plays an important role in the appearance of oral cavity and other lesions in patients with BD.

Isogai E et al. has also suggested that streptococcus infection and etiology of BD were related. Recently, they applied heat shock to *Streptococcus sanguis* infected mice to demonstrate infection with *Streptococcus sanguis* was associated with BD. *Streptococcus sanguis* strain BD 113–20 was inoculated in the oral cavity of germ free mice and the effect of heat shock was examined. Colonization was persistent, inflammatory cytokines were detected in oral inflammatory sites, and ocular lesions, and systemic immune response was seen in the heat shock group. Pretreatment of heat shock enhanced the inflammatory response of oral mucosa in the mice [5]. Ohno group also reported *Streptococcus sanguis* infection and neutrophil hypersensitivity in the development of BD in mice. Granulocyte-colony stimulating factor (G-CSF) has a priming activity on neutrophil function. G-CSF alone did not stimulate the respiratory burst, but primes for superoxide production with various stimuli. *Streptococcus sanguis* was infected in oral and sub-mucosal area of G-CSF transgenic mice. There was a clear association between the number of *Streptococcus sanguis* and severity of the disease process. This evidence suggested that bacteria could induce primary mediators of the inflammatory process [6].

It is well known that Hulusi Behçet first described and speculated that the lesions might be from viral infection according to his clinical observations. Later, Sezer FN [7] and Evans AD et al. [8] also reported that BD was caused by viral infection but they did not mention any specific virus probably due to the limits of diagnostic tools at that time.

Table 2   Detection of HSV DNA in various lesions of Behçet's disease by PCR.

Lesions	Groups	n	Positive n (%)	p-value
Saliva	Patients	66	26 (39.4)	< 0.01
	Control (normal healthy)	87	12 (13.8)	
Genital ulcer	Patients	9	6 (66.7)	< 0.01
	Control (normal healthy)	9	0 (0.0)	
EN-like skin lesion	Patients	20	13 (65.0)	< 0.01
	Uninvolved skin of patients	15	5 (33.3)	
	Psoriasis	10	1 (10.0)	
	Control subjects	20	4 (20.0)	
Intestinal ulcer	Patients	7	7 (100.0)	< 0.001
	Control (Crohn's disease)	13	2 (15.4)	

Due to the development of polymerase chain reaction (PCR) technique, research related to viral infection became active. In 1991, Studd M et al. first reported that HSV-1 DNA was highly detected in blood cells of patients with recurrent oral ulcers and patients with BD compared to controls using PCR [9]. Our study group also confirmed that in the saliva of patients with BD, HSV DNA was detected statistically higher by PCR. Of 66 DNA preparations from the saliva of the patients, 26 (39.4%) showed the HSV DNA band. This contrasts with 12 of 87 preparations (13.8%) from healthy controls [10] (Fig. 1). In genital ulcers of BD patients, all 9 patients showed the HSV DNA band. As for the control, nine episiotomized tissues did not show any HSV DNA band [11]. Also, in intestinal ulcers of BD patients, all 7 patients showed the HSV DNA band. As for the control, 13 patients with Crohn's disease showed 2 positive HSV DNA [12] (Figs. 2,3). In erythema-nodosum-like lesion, 13 out of 20 patients showed positive HSV DNA (Table 2).

Based on the above-mentioned results, we induced BD-like symptoms inoculated by HSV in ICR mice. 258 mice were inoculated with HSV in a scratched earlobe twice in 4 week intervals and followed for the next 16 weeks. About 30% of inoculated mice showed BD-like symptoms, accompanied more than two symptoms in one mouse [13] (Fig. 4). Strangely, when we tried this with hairless mice, none of the 23 mice showed any BD-like symptoms. We thought that major histocompatibility complex (MHC) could be involved in development of BD symptoms. We then applied HSV to several inbred mice, such as B10.BR (H-2k), B10.RIII (H-2r), C57BL/6 (H-2b), C3H/He (H-2k), Balb/c (H-2d), which have different types of MHC. BD-like symptoms developed in 40–50% of B10.BR, B10.RIII and C57BL/6 strains, but in only 2% of C3H/He and Balb/c (Table 3). B10.BR and C3H/He strains had a common haplotype (H-2k), but the rate of manifestation was different. Therefore, we concluded that MHC is not directly correlated with development of BD-like symptoms [14].

Kim YC et al. tried to determine if herpes infection regulated the expression of cell adhesion molecules in cultured human dermal microvascular endothelial cells(HDMEC) and if it regulated T lymphocytes binding to HDMEC. The expression of intracellular adhesion molecule 1 (ICAM-1), vascular cell adhesion molecule-1 (VCAM-1), or E-selectin on HDMEC increased after treatment with HSV-1, HSV-2

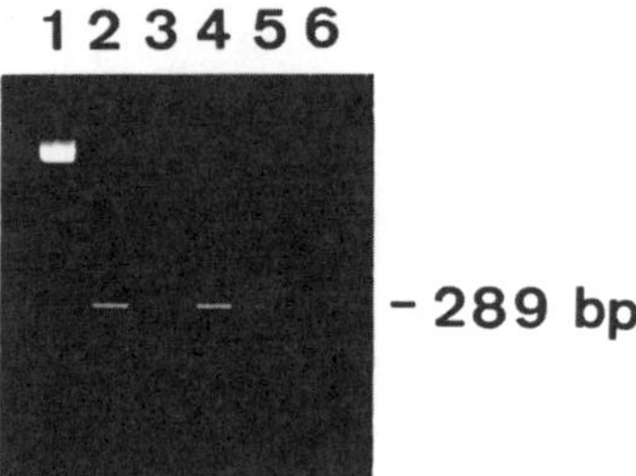

Figure 1 Electrophoresis of PCR amplified HSV DNA in saliva of patients with Behçet's disease. lane 1; 123 DNA ladder as size marker, lane 2; positive control, lane 3; negative control, lane 4–6; patients sample.

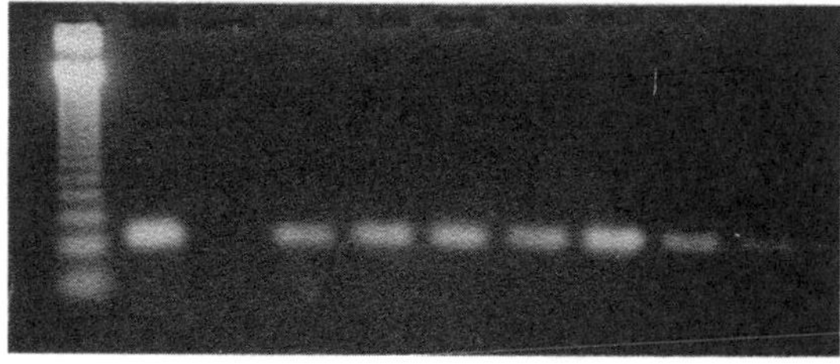

Figure 2 PCR reveals HSV DNA in Behçet's disease patients with intestinal ulcer. M; 123 DNA ladder as size marker, C; positive control, N; negative control, 1–7; patients sample.

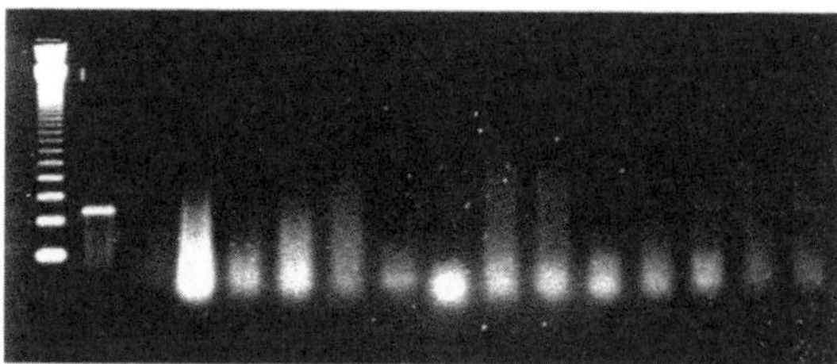

Figure 3 PCR reveals HSV DNA in patients with intestinal Crohn's disease from deparaffinized tissue.

or measles virus on HDMEC. The increased binding of T-lymphocyte after treatment with HSV-1 was significantly decreased by co-incubating with anti-ICAM-1 antibody or with anti-ICAM-1, anti-VCAM-1 and E-selectin antibody simultaneously [15] (Fig. 5,6).

Seonghyang Sohn et al.

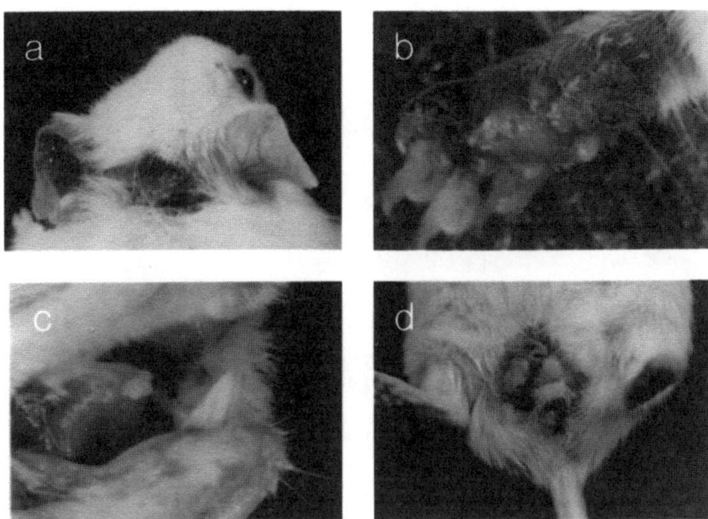

Figure 4 BD-like symptoms; a. earlobe and scruff ulcer, b. arthritis, c. oral ulcer, d. genital ulcer.

Table 3 The number of Behçet's disease-like symptomatic mice and strains after ear-lobe inoculation with 1.0×10^6 p.f.u. of HSV.

					No. (%)
Strain	B10.BR	B10.RIII	C57BL/6	C3H/He	Balb/c
BD Symptoms	27 (50.0)	24 (49.0)	12 (40.0)	1 (2.0)	1 (2.2)
Death	5 (9.3)	6 (12.2)	4 (13.3)	2 (4.0)	3(6.7)
Normal	22 (40.7)	19 (38.8)	14 (46.7)	46 (94.0)	41(91.1)
Total	54 (100)	49 (100)	30 (100)	49 (100)	45 (100)

BD: Behçet's Disease-like.
B10.BR, B10.RIII, C57BL/6 and C3H/He strains were bred to 4 weeks old in SPF animal facility, then transferred to conventional clean facility.

Famciclovir, an antiviral compound, was administered for the treatment of lesions, such as oral, genital, skin ulcer, and eye involvement, in the HSV-induced BD mouse model. Famciclovir improved these BD-like symptoms (Fig. 7). Administration of Famciclovir from the day of lesion occurrence was effective in 40% of BD-like symptoms (Table 4). Specifically, Famciclovir treated BD-like mice did not have a recurrence of oral and genital ulcers. Pretreatment or concurrent treatment of Famciclovir with HSV injection did not affect the incidence of development of BD-like symptoms. After Famciclovir administration, IL-2 expression correlated with the recurrence of BD-like symptoms. This may indicate the possible role of immune responses combined with bacterial or viral infection in development and activation of BD [16].

The Lehner group has suggested that heat shock protein (HSP) plays a critical role in etiology of BD. Stress proteins or HSP are immunoreactive proteins found in

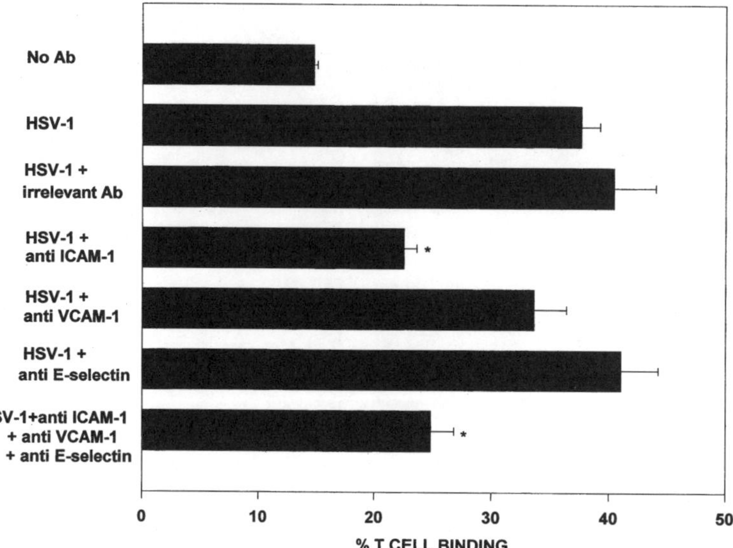

Figure 5 Effect of anti-cell adhesion molecules antibody on T-lymphocytes-HDMEC binding. The increased binding of T-lymphocyte after treatment with HSV-1 was significantly decreased by co-incubating with anti-ICAM-1 antibody or by co-incubating with anti-ICAM-1 antibody, anti-VCAM-1 antibody and anti-E-selectin antibody simultaneously.

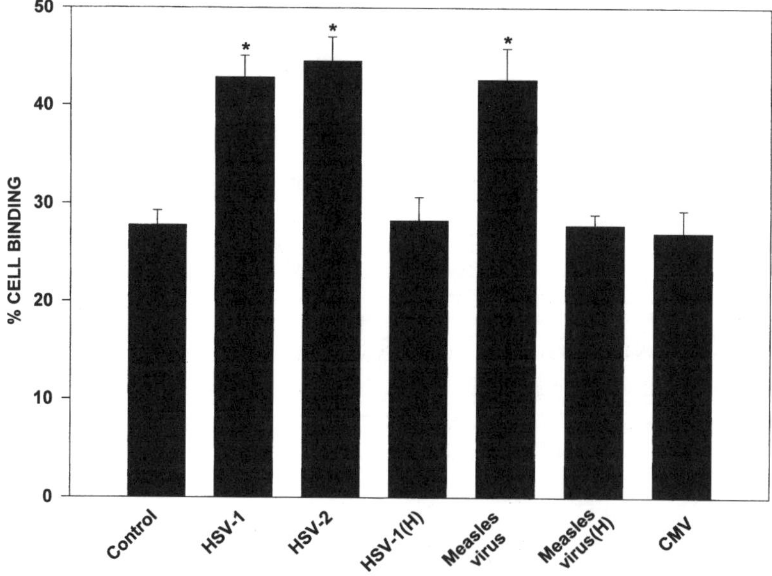

Figure 6 Effect of HSV and measles virus on T-lymphocytes-HDMEC adherence. HDMEC were treated with HSV-1, heat-inactivated HSV-1, HSV-2, measles virus, and CMV for 4 h and co-incubated with ^{51}Cr labeled T-lymphocytes. The binding of T-lymphocytes increased after treatment with HSV-1, HSV-2, and measles virus, but did not increase significantly after treatment with heat-inactivated HSV-1 or CMV.

Seonghyang Sohn et al.

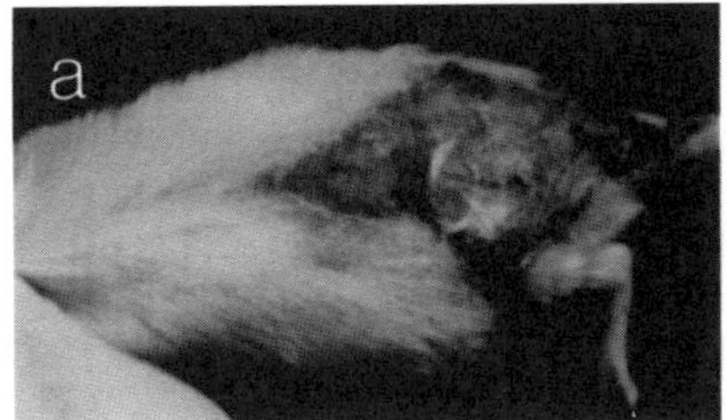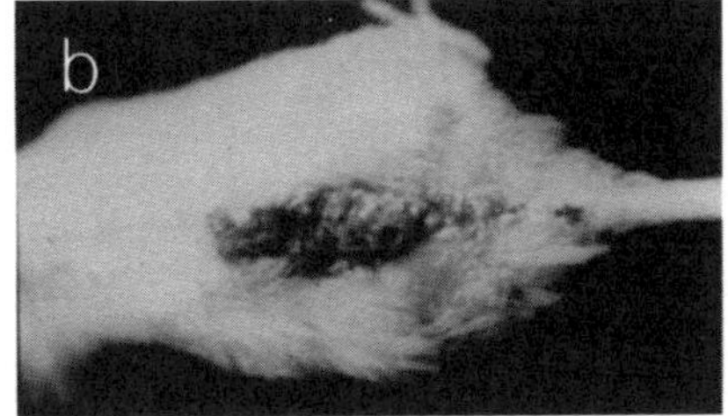

Figure 7   Famciclovir administration to BD-like mice. After Famciclovir administration, 40% of BD-like mice were improved. a. before the administration, b. after the Administration.

Table 4   Famciclovir efficacy in herpes simplex virus inoculated symptomatic ICR mice

	Single symptom n=26 (%)	BD symptom n=25 (%)
Initial improvement	20 (77.0)	22 (88.0)
Recurrence	5 (19.2)	12 (48.0)
Actual improvement	15 (57.7)	10 (40.0)
No change	1 (3.8)	–
Deterioration	1 (3.8)	–

Improvement after the famciclovir treatment occurred for bullae and skin crusting, as well as for oral, genital, and skin ulcers, and eye involvement. Recurrent symptoms after famciclovir treatment consisted of skin ulcers at the same or different site, and eye involvement.

microorganism and animal tissues. Besides heat, stress proteins are also induced by anoxia, heavy metals, H_2O_2, and viruses. The rationale for investigation of HSP in the pathogenesis of Behçet's disease is that 4 species of streptococci (*Streptococcus sanguis, pyogenes, faecalis, salivarius*) have been implicated in the etiology of BD. Microbial (Mycobacterium) HSP 65 kD has homology with human HSP 60 kD. Human 60 kD HSP derived peptide 336–351 induced clinical and/or histological uveitis in 80% of subcutaneous immunized rats. The single symptom of this animal model is the clinical symptom, uveitis [17]. If HSP could induce BD symptoms (at least two symptoms in one animal) in rats, it could very clearly explain the etiology of BD because HSP could explain the hypotheses of streptococcal infection, viral infection, and even environmental pollutants. However, HSP was not enough even though it has obvious roles in inducting BD symptoms, specifically, eye symptom.

What is the other factor contributing to the induction for BD by combinational reaction with HSP? When macrophage knockout with liposome-encapsulated clodronate, the incidence of BD was lowered compared to no-knockout group in ICR mice. Macrophage knockout group expressed Th2 cytokine, IL-4. Th2 cytokine, IL-4 and IL-10 have important roles in the improving BD symptoms in HSV-induced mouse model [18]. Balancing Th1 and Th2 cytokine might be part of its role in induction of BD.

CONCLUSION

From the above, we can conclude that HSV is one of the etiological triggering factors in pathogenesis of BD. However, the role of HSV in pathogenesis of BD does not rule out the streptococcal infection. Also, the induction of BD could possibly by not only cause streptococcal infection and HSV infection but also other factors such as environmental pollution or standard of living.

REFERENCES

1. Kaneko F, Kaneda T, Ohnishi O, Kishiyama K, Takashima I, Hukuda H, Kado Y, Endo M. 1978. Behçet's syndrome and infection allergy. (1) Detection of chronic infectious foci and immune responses to bacterial vaccines in vivo and in vitro. *Japanese J Allergology* 1978; 113: 303.

2. Kaneko F, Miura Y, Kishiyama K, Takashima I, Fukuda H, Kado Y, Endo M. Behçet's syndrome and infection allergy. In Gonzales-Ochoa A, DomingueZ-Soto L, Ortiz Y eds. *International Congress Series No. 451*, Dermatology. Excepta Medica, Amsterdam, Oxford, Princeton, 1977, 162–165.

3. Kaneko F, Takahashi Y, Muramatsu Y, Miura Y. Immunological studies on aphthous ulcer and erythema nodosum-like eruptions in Behçet's disease. *British J Dermatology* 1985; 113: 303–312.

4. Kaneko F, Suzuki M, Suzuki S. Behçet's disease and streptoccoci: Could *Streptococcal salivarius* play an important role in the mechanism of aphthous ulceration. In: O'Duffy JD, Kokmen E, Editors, *Proceedings of the Fifth International Conference on Behçet's disease.* New York: Merkel Dekker, 1989; 427–434.

5. Isogai E, Isogai H, Yokota K, Oguma K, Kimura K, Kubota T, Fujii N, Kotake S, Yoshikawa K, Ohno S. Experimental model for Behçet's disease in gnotobiotic mice infected with *Streptococcus sanguis*. *9th International Congress on Behçet's disease.* p.133, 2000, Seoul.

6. Isogai E, Kokai Y, Isogai H, Yokota K, Oguma K, Ishihara M, Ohno S. Mucosal infection of *Streptococcus sanguis* in granulocyte colony-stimulating factor transgenic mice-microbiological model for Behçet's disease. *9th International Congress on Behçet's disease.* p.138, 2000, Seoul.

7. Sezer FN. The isolation of a virus as cause of Behçet's disease: The isolation of a virus as the cause of Behçet's disease. *Am J Ophthalmol* 1953; 36: 301–15.

8. Evans AD, Pallis CA, Spillane JD. Involvement of the nervous system in Behçet's syndrome: report of three cases and isolation of virus. *Lancet* 1957. 2: 349–53.

9. Studd M, McCance DJ, Lehner T. Detection of HSV-1 DNA in patients with Behçet's syndrome and in patients with recurrent oral ulcers by the polymerase chain reaction. *J. Med Microbiol* 1991; 34: 39–43.

10. Lee S, Bang D, Cho YH, Lee ES, Sohn S. Polymerase chain reaction reveals herpes simplex virus DNA in saliva of patient with Behçet's disease. *Arch Dermatol Res* 1996; 288: 179–183.

11. Bang D, Cho YH, Choi H-J, Lee S, Sohn S, ES Lee. Detection of herpes simplex virus DNA by polymerase chain reaction in genital ulcer of patients with Behçet's disease. *7th International Conference on Behçet's disease.* p.74–6, 1996, Tunis.

Seonghyang Sohn et al.

12. Lee ES, Lee S, Bang D, Sohn S. Herpes simplex virus detection by polymerase chain reaction in intestinal ulcer of patients with Behçet's disease. *7th International Conference on Behçet's disease.* p.71–3, 1996, Tunis.

13. Sohn S, Lee ES, Bang D. Lee S. Behçet's disease-like symptom induced by herpes simplex virus in ICR mice. *European Journal of Dermatology*, 1998; 8: 21–23.

14. Sohn S, Lee ES, Lee S. The correlation of MHC haplotype and development of Behçet's disease-like symptoms induced by herpes simplex virus in several inbred mouse strains. *J Dermatol Sci.* 2001; 26:173–81.

15. Kim YC, Bang D, Lee S, Lee KH. The effect of herpes virus infection on the expression of cell adhesion molecules on cultured human dermal microvascular endothelial cells. *J Dermatol Sci* 2000; 24: 38–47.

16. Sohn S, Bang D, Lee E-S, Kwo HJ, Lee SI, Lee S. Experimental Studies of Antiviral Agent-Famciclovir in Behçet's Disease Symptoms of ICR Mice. *Br J Dermatol* 2001 145:799–804

17. Stanford MR, Kasp E, Whiston R, Hasan A, Todryk S, Shinnick T, Mizushima Y, Dumonde DC, van der Zee R, Lehner T. Heat shock protein peptides reactive in patients with Behçet's disease are uveitogenic in Lewis rats. *Clin Exp Immunol.* 1994; 97: 226–31.

18. Sohn S, Lee ES, Kwon HJ, Lee SI, Bang D, Lee S. Expression of Th2 cytokines decreased the development and improved the Behçets disease-like symptoms induced by herpes simplex virus in mice. *J Infect Dis.* 2001; 183: 1180–6.

THOMAS LEHNER

13. The Role of Heat Shock Proteins in Behçet's Disease

ABSTRACT

The aetiology of Behçet's disease (BD) has been associated with some strains of *Streptococcus sanguis* and Herpes simplex virus. Heat shock protein (HSP) is a common microbial agent and has significant homology with human cellular HSP. The evidence in favour of HSP as an aetiological factor in BD was initially based on finding significantly increased T cell proliferative responses and B cell antibodies to defined HSP65 epitopes in patients with BD. These peptide epitopes induce uveitis in Lewis rats, when administered by the oral mucosal or systemic route. Furthermore, the stress response MICA gene shares nucleotide sequences with the human HSP70 promoter and is in linkage disequilibrium with HLA-B51. During active disease, cytokine and chemokine networks are polarised towards the TH1 cytokines. The evidence from the studies of HSP, MICA gene and γδ T cells has converged towards the concept that the multi-system immunopathology of BD is generated by an over-reaction to microbial stress proteins.

KEYWORDS   Behçet's disease; heat shock proteins; γδ T cells.

INTRODUCTION

The aetiology of BD has been associated with a variety of microorganisms,especially Herpes simplex virus and *Streptococcus sanguis*. A common microbial agent may be involved, such as heat shock protein (HSP) which shows significant homology with human cellular HSP. The evidence in favour of HSP as an aetiological factor and in the pathogenesis of BD will be reviewed. The concept will be developed that the multisystem immunopathology of BD is caused by an over-reaction to microbial stress proteins.

Streptococcus sanguis or its cross-reactivity with oral epithelial antigens has been implicated in the aetiology of recurrent oral ulcers [1–3] and *S. sanguis, S. pyogenes, S, faecalis* and *S. salivarius* in the aetiology of BD [4, 5]. The *S. sanguis* found in lesions of patients with BD were uncommon serotypes [6]. Significant IgA and to a lesser extent IgG antibodies to these streptococci (KTH-1 to 3) were found in patients with BD [7]. *S. sanguis* stimulated T cell proliferation, IL-6 production and upregulation of mRNA of IL-2 and IFNγ [8, 9]. Furthermore, *S. sanguis* found in BD cross-reacted with oral mucosal antigens and this was accounted for by shared homology between the microbial and human 65kD heat shock protein [7]. This is also consistent with early autoimmune findings in BD and recurrent oral ulceration [10, 11].

The number of strains of streptococci implicated in the aetiology of BD and the cross-reactivity with oral mucosal antigens raised the hypothesis [7] that a common antigen, such as stress or heat shock protein (HSP) found in most Gram-positive bacteria [12] might account for these diverse observations. Indeed, Western blot showed cross-reactivity between these streptococci and the HSP65, as well as significant increases in IgA and IgG antibodies to HSP65 in sera from patients with BD [7]. Although stimulation of PBMC with HSP65 yielded high stimulation indices in BD (10.9 ± 1.8), this was not significantly different from healthy controls, disease controls or patients with recurrent oral ulcers [13]. HSP from one bacterial species shows considerable homology with that of other bacterial species, so enhanced immunity may be boosted naturally by intercurrent infections that have been implicated in BD.

T AND B CELL EPITOPE MAPPING OF HSP

T cell epitope mapping (Fig. 1) identified 4 peptides derived from the sequence of the 65kD HSP [13] which stimulate specifically $\gamma\delta^+$ T cells from patients with BD [14]. These peptides (111–125, 154–172, 219–233 and 311–325) showed significant homology with the corresponding peptides derived from the human 60kD HSP [13]. The B cell epitopes within mycobacterial HSP65 or human HSP60 overlapped with the T cell epitopes and both IgG and IgA antibodies were identified [15]. Among the 4 T and B cell epitopes, peptide 336–351 or microbial HSP65 (311–325) is significantly associated with BD in Britain [13, 14], Japan [16] and Turkey [17]. HSP60/65 was also found to be significantly increased in the epidermal cells of skin lesions in BD [18], and antibodies to HSP65 were raised in the cerebrospinal fluid from patients with neurological manifestations of BD [19]. Thus, there is an increasing body of evidence to suggest the involvement of HSP65 and specific epitopes within this molecule in the pathogenesis of BD.

Further T cell epitope mapping within the HSP65 molecule revealed that peptide 91–105 is specific in stimulating T cell proliferation in patients with recurrent oral ulcers [20]. This epitope is separated only by 5 residues from the BD-specific peptide 111–125. Furthermore, the epitope responsible for adjuvant arthritis in Lewis rats (p.180–188) is found between two BD epitopes (p.154–179 and p.219–233). These findings raise the possibility that adjuvant arthritis in rats may be more relevant as an

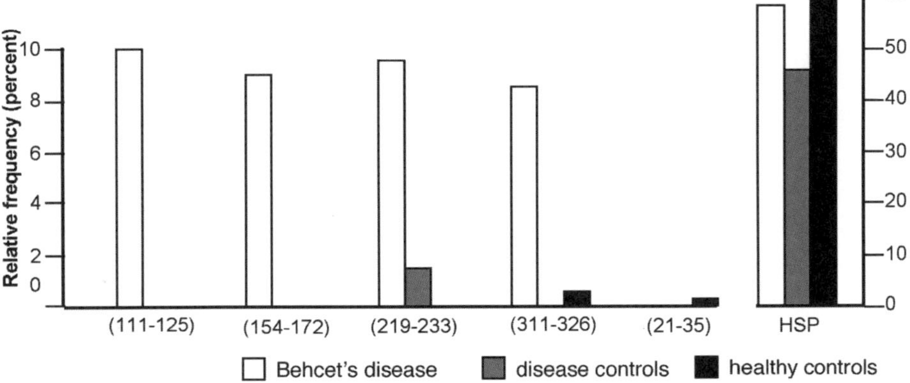

Figure 1 Relative frequency of short term cell lines (STCL) yielding stimulation indices ≥ 3 with 4 selected peptides, heat shock protein (HSP) and a control peptide.

animal model of BD arthritis than that of rheumatoid arthritis which is more distant (p.241–265), especially if conformational epitopes are involved.

It is remarkable that although ROU is the only consistent feature of BD, the T cell proliferative response to peptide 91–105 is lost in BD. Thus, T cells from patients with ROU respond only to peptide 91–105, whereas patients with BD, still manifesting ROU, loose their reactivity to this peptide and develop a responses especially to peptide 336–351. The intramolecular switch in HSP65 from aa 91–105 to 336–351 is therefore of great significance and deserves further attention. Peptide 91–105 has been subjected to further studies [21] and this revealed that the critical residues are found in the carboxy terminal part of peptide 91–105 (residues Leu 98, Arg 100, Arg 104 and Asn 105).

PATHOGENICITY OF HSP65 PEPTIDES

The potential pathogenicity of these peptides in inducing some of the manifestations of BD was then tested in Lewis rats. Subcutaneous immunization with any of the 4 peptides but especially with peptide 336–351 and adjuvants elicited uveitis in about 80% of Lewis rats [22, 23]. A mucosal model of induction of uveitis was then developed in rats by oral or nasal administration of p336–351 without an adjuvant [24], and this is consistent with the onset of oral ulceration in more than 90% of patients with BD. Mucosal induction of experimental uveitis appears to be mediated by $CD4^+$ T cells, whereas suppression is induced by $CD8^+$ T cells or IL-4 [24]. This finding is consistent with peptide 336–351 eliciting IL-12, a TH1 cytokine from $CD4^+$ T cells, whereas $CD8^+$ T cells secrete cytokines which suppress TH1 cell function [25].

ADJUVANT EFFECT OF HSP

Microbial HSP65 and HSP70 function as potent stimulators of the 3 CC chemokines, RANTES, MIP-1α and MIP-1β but not MCP-1 (Fig. 2) [26]. The chemokines are

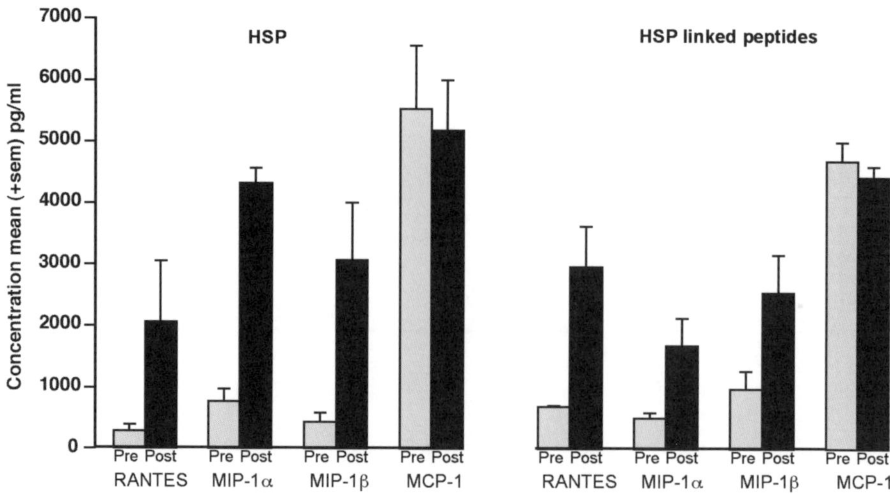

Figure 2   The effect of targeted iliac lymph node immunization with the mycobacterial 65 or 70 kD HSP, 3 times at monthly intervals in rhesus macaques, on the concentration of CC chemokines (pg/ml) before and 1 month after the 3rd immunization.

generated to a comparable extent, irrespective of whether the HSP is empty (i.e. ATP-treated) or loaded with a peptide (Fig. 2). The function of these chemokines is to attract immature dendritic cells, macrophages, T and B cells [27–31]. It is therefore not surprising that HSP65 and HSP70 act as systemic [32, 33], as well as mucosal adjuvants [26]. HSP65 and HSP70 are the only known reagents to modulate both systemic and mucosal immunity and this property might be important in BD which is one of a few multisystem diseases with major mucosal and systemic manifestations. An important issue, however needs to be resolved, that is whether the microbial HSP cross-reacting with human HSP is adequate to account for the immunopathogenesis of BD or if there is a peptide within the pocket of HSP that is specific for BD. It is noteworthy that HSP70 acts as molecular chaperone in folding, unfolding and trans-location of proteins and peptides [34]. It is also significant that HSP70 is one of the few external reagents that can translocate antigens into the class I pathway, thereby inducing TH1-type immune responses [35].

Investigation of HSP has suffered in the past from a failure to identify the corresponding receptors. This has been rectified very recently, by the report that human HSP60 binds to CD14 [36] which functions as an innate receptor on macrophages and neutrophils. However, microbial HSP70 utilises the CD40 receptor [37] which is a costimulatory molecule on dendritic cells, macrophages and B cells and is critical in the interactions with the CD40 ligand, especially in CD8[+] T cell responses [38, 39]. Interaction between HSP70 and CD40 costimulatory molecules activates CC chemokines and may function as a bridge between innate and adaptive immunity [37].

Thomas Lehner

Further support for HSP involvement in BD comes from the finding that HSP65 and HSP70 stimulates γδ T cells to proliferate [40–42] and to generate the 3 CC chemokines [26]. γδ⁺ T cells are present in up to 10% of circulating blood of healthy individuals and are usually either CD3⁺ CD4⁻ CD8⁻ or CD8⁺ T cells. An increased number of γδ⁺ T cells are found in the intestinal and female genital tracts. The proportion of γδ T cells is significantly increased in BD [43–46] and this is consistent with HSP65 and/or HSP70 stimulating γδ T cells [40–42, 26]. This subset differs from αβ T cells in that it is not HLA restricted, and MICA molecules can present peptides to γδ T cells [47]. HSP peptides specific for BD stimulate γδ T cells to proliferate [14]. Because of the high specificity of these peptides for BD, stimulation of the T cell proliferative response with the peptides can be used as a laboratory diagnostic test for BD. *S. sanguis* also stimulates γδ T cells to generate IL-2 and IFNγ mRNA [10]. We suggest that γδ T cells play an essential role in the immunopathogenesis of BD, as they have been consistently found to be increased in BD [43–46]. Stimulation of γδ T cells with microbial HSP or their constitutive peptides, coupled with the capacity of MICA gene product to present peptides to γδ T cells [47], enhances the significance of this subset of T cells in BD. The precise function of γδ T cells in BD needs to be determined but they may initiate mucosal ulceration through their capacity (a) to generate TH1 or TH2 cytokines [48], (b) to function as killer cells [49], (c) by mediating expression of a keratinocyte growth factor (50), (d) by activating αβ T cells [51] and (e) by generating CC chemokines [26].

MICROBIAL STRESS-INDUCED INNATE IMMUNITY MAY DRIVE ADAPTIVE IMMUNITY IN BD

The evidence from a number of laboratories worldwide has converged on to the concept that the multi-system pathology in BD might be initiated by microbial stress, activating HSP and the MICA cell stress response gene in epithelial cells. Indeed, MICA contains heat shock elements defined in HSP70 genes and share nucleotide sequences homologous with the human HSP70 promoter [50]. Thus, microbial stress may activate HSP and MICA, and induce in genetically predisposed individuals a cascade of cytokines and chemokines to stimulate innate immune responses. The receptor for human HSP60 has been recently identified as CD14 [36], whereas the microbial HSP70 utilises the CD40 receptor [37].

CD14 receptors are found on macrophages and neutrophils, whereas CD40 receptors have a wider distribution, on macrophages, dendritic cells, B cells and endothelial cells. These cells are stimulated to generate an array of cytokines and chemokines that will elicit increased vascular permeability, acute phase proteins (including CRP, factor B and C9), and chemoattraction of mononuclear cells and neutrophils (Fig. 3).

Innate immunity may drive adaptive immunity with specific CD4, CD8, γδ T cell and B cell responses and polarization towards the TH1-type of cytokines. Overall, the recognition of interactions between HSP, MICA and γδ⁺ T cells in the immunopathogenesis of BD raises the provocative hypothesis that BD might be a disease generated

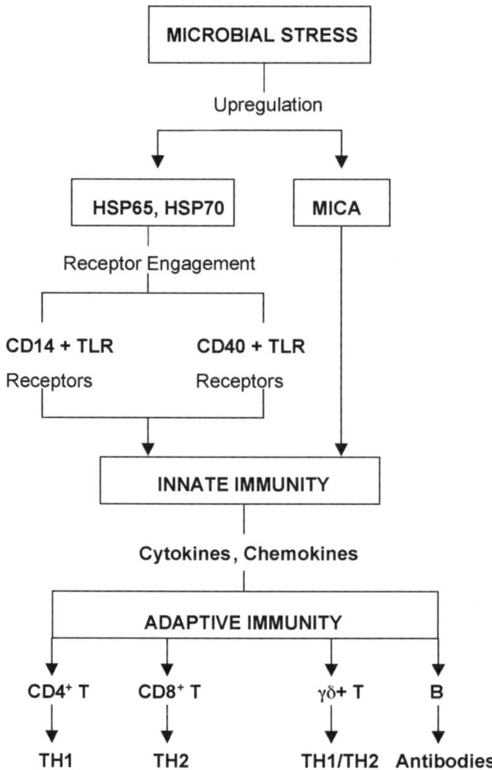

Fig. 3   The potential role of HSP in the immunopathognesis of Behçet's Disease.

by over-reaction to microbial stress proteins. Essential elements in future research are (a) To determine if the BD-HSP specific peptide can suppress the development of uveitis not only in rats but also in humans. To this end a clinical phase I/II trial has been launched. (b) To identify the critical cytokines and chemokines that are responsible for maintaining disease activity. (c) To find out if HSP carry another peptide(s) specific for BD in addition to the integral HSP defined peptides.

CONCLUSIONS

Behçet's disease affects muco-cutaneous, occular, central nervous and joint tissues. The aetiology of BD has been associated with a variety of microorganisms,especially Herpes simplex virus and some strains of *Streptococcus sanguis*. A common microbial agent may be involved, such as heat shock protein (HSP) which has significant homology with human cellular HSP. The evidence in favour of HSP as an aetiological factor in BD is based on the following findings. (a) T cell proliferative responses and B cell antibodies are significantly increased to defined HSP65 epitopes in patients

                                                        Thomas Lehner

with BD in Britain, Japan and Turkey. (b) γδ T cells are significantly increased in BD and HSP65 or 70 upregulates γδ T cells. (c) The HSP-peptide determinants defined in patients with BD elicit uveitis in Lewis rats when administered by the oral mucosal or systemic route. (d) HSP65 or HSP70 modulate both mucosal and systemic immunity, by virtue of stimulating the production of chemokines and cytokines. (e) The MICA gene is a cell stress response gene and shares nucleotide sequences with the human HSP70 promoter. A significant association has been found between BD and the MICA6 or MICA9 allele which is in linkage disequilibrium with HLA-B51 The cytokine and chemokine networks are stimulated with polarisation towards the TH1 cytokines during active disease. The evidence from the studies of HSP, MICA gene and γδ T cells has converged towards the concept that the multi-system immunopathology of BD is generated by an over-reaction to microbial stress proteins.

REFERENCES

1. Graykowski, E.A., Barile, M.F., Lee, W/B/ and Stanley, H.R. *J Am. Med. Assoc.* 196:637–644, 1996.
2. Donatsky, O. *Scand. J. Dent. Res.* 83:111–119, 1975.
3. Wilton, J.M.A. and Lehner, T. *J. Dent. Res.* 47:1001, 1968.
4. Kaneko, F., Takahashi, Y., Muramatsu, Y., Miura, Y. *Br. J. Dermatol.* 113:303–12, 1985.
5. Mizushima, Y. *J. Rheumatol.* 16:506–11, 1989.
6. Isogai, E., Ohno, S., Takehashi, K. et al. *Bifidobact Microflora* 9, 27–41, 1990.
7. Lehner, T., Lavery, E., Smith, R., van der Zee R., Mizushima, Y., Shinnick, T. *Infect. Immun.* 59:1434–41, 1991.
8. Hirohata, S., Oka, H. and Mizushima, Y. *Cell. Immunol.* 140:410–419, 1992.
9. Mochizuki, M., Suzuki, N., Takeno, M. et al. *Eur. J. Immunol.* 24:1536–1543, 1994.
10. Shimizu, T., Katsuta, Y. and Oshima, Y. *Ann. Rheum. Dis.* 24:494, 1965.
11. Lehner, T. *Br. Med. J.* I:465–467, 1967.
12. Thole, J.E.R., Hindersson, R.P., de Bruyn, J. et al. *Microb. Pathol.* 4, 71–83, 1988.
13. Pervin, K., Childerstone, A., Shinnick, T. et al. *J. Immunol.* 151:1–10, 1993.
14. Hasan, A., Fortune, F., Wilson, A. et al. *Lancet.* 347:789–794, 1996.
15. Direskeneli, H., Hasan, A., Shinnick, T. et al. *Scand. J. Immunol.* 43:464–471, 1996.
16. Kaneko, S., Suzuki, N., Yamashita, N. et al. *Clin. Exp. Immunol.* 108:204–212, 1997.
17. Direskeneli, H., Eksloglu-Demiralp, E., Yavuz, T. et al. *J. Rhematol.* 708–713, 2000.
18. Ergun, T., Ince, U., Demiralp, E. et al. 8th International Congress on Behçet's Disease. Reggio Emilia, P52, 1998.
19. Tasci, B., Direskeneli, H., Serdaroglu, P. et al. *Clin. Exp. Immunol.* 113:100–104, 1998.
20. Hasan, A., Childerstone, A., Pervin, K. et al. *Clin. Exp. Immunol.* 99:392–397, 1995.
21. Hasan, A., Wilson, A., Shinnick, T., Mizushima, Y., van der Zee, R., Stanford, M. and Lehner, T.. *Clin.Exp.Immunol.* (in press) 2001.
22. Stanford, M.R., Kasp, E., Whiston, R. et al. *Clin. Exp. Immunl.* 97:226–231, 1994.
23. Uchio, E., Stanford, M., Hasan, A. et al. *Exp. Eye. Res.* 16:174–180, 1998.
24. Hu, W., Hasan, A., Wilson, A. et al. *Eur. J. Immunol.* 28:2444–2455, 1998.
25. Sakane, T., Suzuki, N. and Taneko, M. 8th International Congress on Behçet's Disease. Reggio Emilia, L14, 1998.
26. Lehner, T., Bergmeier, L.A., Wang, Y. et al. *Eur. J. Immunol.* 30:594–603, 2000.
27. Murphey, P.M.. *Annu. Rev. Immunol.* 12:593–633, 1994.
28. Mcurer, R., Van Riper, G., Feeney, W. et al. *J. Exp. Med.* 178:1913–1921, 1993.

29. Kim, J.J., Nottingham, L.K., Sin, J.I. et al. *J. Clin. Invest.* 102:1112–1124, 1998.

30. Schall, T.J., Bacon, K., Camp, R.D. et al. *J. Exp. Med.* 177:1821–1826, 1993.

31. Dieu, M.C., Vanbervliet, B., Vicari, A. et al. *J. Exp. Med.* 188:378–386, 1998.

32. Lussow, A.R., Barrios, C., van Embden, J. et al. *Eur. J. Immunol.* 21:2297–2302, 1991.

33. Perraut, R., Lussow, A.R., Gavoille, S. et al. *Clin. Exp. Immunol.* 93:382–386, 1993.

34. Pilon, M., and Schekman, R. *Cell.* 97:679–682, 1999.

35. Fujihara, S.M. and Nadler, S.G. *The EMBO J.* 18, 411–419, 1999.

36. Kol, A., Lightman, A.H., Finberg, R.W., Libby, P. and Kurt-Jones, E.A. *J. Immunol.* 164: 13–17, 2000.

37. Wang, Y., Kelly, C., Kartunen, J. et al. *Immunity.* (In press) 2001.

38. Ridge, J.P., Di Rose, F. and Matzinger, P. *Nature.* 393:474–478, 1998.

39. Bennett, S.R.M., Carbone, F.R., Karamalis, F. et al. *Nature.* 393:478–480, 1998.

40. Haregewoin, A., Soman, G., Hom, R.C. and Finberg, R.W.. *Nature.* 340:309–312, 1989.

41. Born, W., Hall, L., Dallas, A. et al. *Science.* 249:67, 1990.

42. Kaur, I., Voss, S.D., Gupta, R.S. et al. *J. Immunol.* 150:2046–2055, 1993.

43. Fortune,. F., Walker. J, and Lehner, T. *Clin. Exp. Immunol.* 82:326–332, 1990.

44. Suzuki, Y., Hoshi, K., Matsuda, T., and Mizushima, Y. *J. Rheumatol.* 19:588–592, 1992.

45. Hamzaoui, K., Hamzaoui, A. and Hentati, F. et al. *J. Rheumatol.* 21:2301–2306, 1994.

46. Yamashita, N., Kaneoka, H., Kaneko, S. et al. *Clin. Exp. Immunol.* 107:241–247, 1997.

47. Steinle, A., Groh, V., and Spies, T. *Proc. Natl. Acad. Sci. USA.* 95:12510–12515, 1998.

48. Ferrick, D.A., Schrenzel, M.D., Mulvania, T. et al. *Nature.* 373:255–257, 1995.

49. Munk, E., Gatrill, A.J.. and Kaufmann, S.H.E. *J. Immunol.* 145:2434–2439, 1990.

50. Boismenu, R and Havran, R. *Science.* 266:1253–1255, 1994.

51. Kaufmann, S., H., E., Blum, C. and Yamamoto, S. *Proc.Natl.Acad.Sci.USA.* 90:9620–9624, 1993.

 Thomas Lehner

CLAUDIA A. MÜLLER, ILHAN GÜNAYDIN, NICOLE STÜBIGER, HASAN
YAZICI, IZZET FRESKO, CHRISTOS C. ZOUBOULIS, YAEL ADLER, INGE
STEIERT, BERND KURZ, DOROTHEE WERNET, BEATE BRAUN AND INA KÖTTER

14. Association of HLA-B51 Suballeles with Behçet's Disease in Patients of German and Turkish Origin

ABSTRACT

Behçet's disease (BD) is suspected to be triggered by environmental factors like infections in patients with a particular genetic background. Besides an association of BD to HLA-B51, a strong association to the transmembrane MICA allele A6 and the extracellular MICA*009 have beeen described. Although the contribution of the HLA-B51 molecule to the overall genetic susceptibility is estimated lower than 20%, HLAB51 seems to be the only relevant pathogenic factor in BD.

KEYWORDS: Behçet's disease; HLA-B51; MICA*009; genetic susceptibility

INTRODUCTION

Behçet's disease (BD), a multisystemic inflammatory disorder with histopathologic features of a leukocytoclastic vasculitis,.is mainly characterized by oral and genital aphthous ulcers, skin lesions (papulopustules, erythema nodosum), uveitis/retinal vasculitis, oligoarthritis, thrombophlebitis or major embolism, vascular aneurysms, gastrointestinal ulcerations, and CNS vasculitis [1]. Behçet's disease is most prevalent in countries along the former "Silk Road" (Mediterranean countries, Middle East, Asia [2]. The prevalence in Turkey is 370/100.000 in Anatolia and 80/100.000 in the European part of the country. In Germany (Berlin) (Zouboulis, personal communication) the estimated prevalence among the Turkish inhabitants is 20,75/100.000, among the Germans 0,55/100.000 (mean 2,26). Disease onset mainly occurs between the age of 20 and 30 in all populations studied so far.

Although the etiology and pathogenesis of BD are still unclear, the disease is suspected to be triggered by environmental factors such as streptococcal or certain

Table 1 Phenotype frequencies of HLA-B51 in patients with Behçet's disease of different world populations.

HLA-Allel	Controls	Patients	X^2	p	Rel. Risk	Ref.
	Japan N=140	Japan N=81				Mizuki et al. 1992
B51	20 (14.3%)	47 (58.0%)	46.47	<0.00005	8.3	
B52	26 (18.6%)	10 (12.3%)				
	Greece N=30	Greece N=31				Mizuki et al. 1997
B51	8 (26.75)	25 (80.6%)	15.78	<0.001	11.46	
B52	0	1 (3.2%)				
	Ireland N=24	Ireland N=96				Kilmartin et al.1997
B51	6 (25.0%)	0	20.3	<0.002	6.3	
B52	0	0				

viral infections in patients with a particular genetic background [3]. Familial aggregation studies suggest a complex inheritance model [4–6]. Among various genetic markers, an association of BD to the HLA-class I molecule HLA-B51 is the most commonly reported [7–10] (Table 1), but also strong associations of BD to the transmembrane MICA allele A6 and the extracellular MICA*009 allele which are inherited centromeric in strong linkage disequilibrium to HLA-B51 have been found [11–14]. Centromeric as well as telomeric regions flanking the HLA-B51 locus including HLA-C or HLA-DR alleles were not observed to show a consistent association with BD (Table 2a,b) [15,16]. Recently, a novel susceptibility locus was claimed to be localised in the telomere of chromosome 6p. [17].

HLA-B51 AND GENETIC PREDISPOSITION

The genetic marker most strongly associated with BD in several ethnic groups is HLA-B51, with a frequency of 50–80% in the different patient groups of Europe and Asia along the Silk route [7–10]. Increased presence of this antigen had an odds ratio of 9.76 (58%, p<0.001) in a group of 33 German BD patients versus 9.13 in 92 Turkish patients (75%, p< 0.001) analysed in our study in comparison to ethnically matched controls (Table 3) [18]. This high prevalence of BD in association to HLA-B51 may hold true only for hospital based patients. In a field study from Turkey, HLA-B51 was present only in 26% of the cases [19]. Thus, it is not yet excluded that HLA-B51 might be a marker of severity of BD rather than susceptibility. In addition, certain Northern Amerindian people who have a high prevalence of HLA-B51 in healthy individuals were not observed to suffer from BD [20]. It has been suggested that the other genetic risk factors present in populations along the Silk Road might be absent among these Amerindians or that causative environmental factors are lacking. In another hypo-

Table 2a Phenotype frequencies of HLA-C alleles among patients with Behçet's disease.

HLA-Allel	Controls	Patients	p	Rel. Risk	Ref.
	Spain N=66	Spain N=56			Sanz et al. 1997
Cw*1602	0	7 (12.5%)	<0.047	20.15 (OR)	
Cw*14	3 (4.5%)	3 (5.3%)			
Cw*15	6 (9.9%)	8 (14.3%)			
	Japan N=96	Japan N=90			Mizuki et al. 1996
Cw*16	0	0			
Cw*14	23 (24.0%)	44 (48.9%)	<0.0005	3.0	
Cw*15	7 (7.3%)	16 (17.8%).	<0.043	2.7	

Table 2b Phenotype frequencies of HLA-DR alleles among patients with Behçet's disease.

HLA-Allel	Controls	Patients	p	Rel. Risk	Ref
	Italian N=28	Italian N=20			Kera et al. 1999
DRB1*11	11 (39.3%)	11 (55.0%)	<0.077		
	Japan N=45	Japan N=79			Mizuki et al. 1992
DRB1*1501	5 (11.1%)	7 (8.9%)	<0.05	0.3	
DRB1*0802	1 (2.2%)	11 (13.9%)	<0.05	4.49	

Table 3 Comparison of German and Turkish patients with Behçet's disease: Frequency of HLA-B51x in patients and controls.

HLA B*51x	All	B*51x pos.	B*51x neg.	Odds ratio	95% confidence interval	p value
GERMAN						
patients	33	19	14			
contols	325	40	285	9,67	4,96 – 18,84	p < 0,001
TURKISH						
patients	92	69	23			
controls	93	23	70	9,13	4,84 – 17,24	p < 0,001

thesis it was postulated that European and Asian populations with BD differ from Amerindians in further genetic markers on the HLA-B51 extended haplotype due to a higher frequency of recombinations within the MHC leading to disruption of further susceptibility loci in linkage to HLA-B51 [2]. Thus, it is still an open debate whether the susceptibility to BD is influenced by HLA-B51 itself or by some other non-HLA genes located around HLA-B in linkage disequilibrium with HLA-B51 [8].

HLA-B51 SUBALLELES AND GENETIC RISK

HLA-B51 has been identified to comprise 29 suballeles at the nucleotide level and 27 subtypes at the protein level (IMGT/HLA Sequence Data Base; *http://www.ebi.ac.uk/ imgt/hla*). It has been reported that HLA-B*5101 is the most frequent suballele (up to 98%) in Japanese, Greek, Spanish, Italian and Arabian patients with BD, followed by HLA-B*5108 [20–1]. In our study, we also performed PCR low- and high-resolution subtyping of the HLA-B*51 locus in order to determine the frequency of HLA-B*51x suballeles in 16 German and 64 Turkish patients and ethnically matched healthy controls (61 German and 23 Turkish healthy controls selected for HLA-B*51x expression) (Table 4). Direct sequencing of overlapping Bw4-related PCR fragments of exon 2 and exon 3 allowed to define all known HLA-B*51x suballeles (B*51011–B*5129). In the German and Turkish controls, a very similar distribution of the HLA-B*51x suballeles was found, with HLA-B*51011 being the most frequent allele in both ethnic control groups (Germans: 93.4%, Turkish: 86.9%) followed by HLA-B*5108 (Germans: 3.5%, Turkish: 10%). HLA-B*5108 showed a slightly higher frequency in both patient groups than in the respective control groups. In addition, HLA-B*5107 present in a healthy German and a Turkish individual was another rare suballele only in the investigated ethnic healthy controls, but not found in the patient groups. All other defined HLA-B*51x suballeles were negative in the German and Turkish healthy and diseased populations. In both patient groups, there was a tendency towards a higher frequency of HLA*B51x homozygous individuals in comparison to their respective controls (Germans: 10% of the patients vs. 2.5% of the controls; Turkish: 27% of the patients vs. 13% of the controls).

The data indicate HLA-*B5101 and HLA-B*5108 as predisposing genes for BD in German and Turkish patients similar to BD cases of other ethnic origin.

HLA-B*5101 and B*5108 share two amino-acid substitutions at position 63 and 67 as the only distinguishable sequence difference in comparison to HLA-B*5201 which is clearly not associated with BD. These amino-acid residues have been suggested to be primarily responsible for the development of BD. The same amino-acid substitutions are present in all other HLA-B*51x suballeles except in B*5107 and

Table 4 Comparison of German and Turkish patients with Behçet disease: Frequencies of HLA-B51 subtype alleles in patients and controls.

HLA-Allel	Controls	Patients	Controls	Patients
	German N=61	German N=16	Turkish N=23	Turkish N=64
B*51011	57 (93.4%)	14 (87.5%)	20 (86.9%)	52 (81.2%)
B*0505	1	0	0	1
B*5107	1	0	1	0
B*5108	2 (3.5%)	2 (14.2%)	2 (10%)	11 (17.1%)

                                              Claudia A. Müller et al.

B*5122. B*5107 shares serin at position 67 with HLA-B*5201 whereas B*5122 carries cystein.

CONCLUSION

Prevalence of BD in different European and Asian populations along the former Silk Road is associated with a significantly elevated frequency of HLA-B*51x. BD in these populations appears to be associated to a common motif of HLA-B*51x rather than to specific suballeles (HLA-B*5101 or B*5108), since no differences in distribution of HLA-*B51x suballeles in both patient and control groups were observed. However, contribution of the HLA-B51 molecule to the overall genetic susceptibility is estimated to be less than 20% [24], since up to 30% of the patients are HLA-B51-negative and since Amerindian populations in spite of a high prevalence of HLA-B51 do not suffer from BD. There may be also other susceptibility genes close or telomer to HLA-B51 on the same haplotype. Although the exact pathogenic mechanism of the HLA-B51 molecule in BD is still unknown, up to now , however, HLA-B51 seems to be the only relevant pathogenic factor in BD [25].

REFERENCES

1. Sakane, T., Takeno, M., Suzuki, N., Inaba, G., *New Engl J Med* 341: 1284–1291, 1999.
2. Verity, D.H., Marr, J.E., Ohno, S., Wallace, G.R., Stanford, M.R., *Tissue Antigens* 54: 213–220, 1999
3. Lehner, T., *Int Rev Immunol* 14: 21–31, 1997.
4. Nishiyama, M., Nakae, K., Kuriyama, T., Hashimoto, M., Hsu, Z.N., *J. Rheumatol.* 29: 743–747, 2002.
5. Nishiyama, M., Nakae, K., Umehara, T., *Jpn. J. Ophthalmol.* 45:313–316, 2001.
6. Mizuki, N., Inoko, H., Mizuki, N., Tanaka, H., Kera, J., Tsuiji, K., Ohno, S., *Invest.Ophthalmol. Vis. Sc.i* 33: 3332–3340, 1992.
7. Mizuki, N., Inoko, H., Ohno, S., *Yonsei Med. J.*; 38: 333–349, 1997.
8. Kilmartin, D.J., Finch, A., Acheson, R.W., *Br. J. Ophthalmol.* 81: 649–653, 1997.
9. Yabuki, K., Ohno, S., Mizuki, N., Ando, H., Tabbara, K.F., Goto, K., Nomura, E., Nakamura, S., Ito, N., Ota, M., Katsuyama, Y., Inoko, H., *Tissue Antigens* 54: 273-277, 1999.
10. Salvarani, C., Boiardi, L., Mantovani, V., Olivieri, I., Ciancio, G., Cantini, F., Salvi, F., Malatesta, R., Molinotti, C., Govoni, M., Trotta, F., Filippini, D., Paolazzi, G., Viggiani, M., *J Rheumatol* 28:1867–1870, 2001.
11. Gonzalez-Escribano, M.F., Rodriguez, M.R., Aguilar, F., Alvarez, A., Sanchez-Roman, J., Nunez-Roldan, A., *Tissue Antigens* 54: 278–281, 1999.
12. Cohen, R., Metzger, S., Nahir, M., Chajek-Shaul, T., *Ann. Rheum. Dis.* 61: 157–160, 2002.
13. Wallace, G.R., Verity, D.H., Delamaine, L.J., Ohno, S., Inoko, H., Ota, M., Mizuki, N., Yabuki, K., Kondiatis, E., Stephens, H.A., Madanat, W., Kanawati, C.A., Stanford, M.R., Vaughan, R.W., *Immunogenetics* 49: 613–617, 1999.
14. Mizuki, N., Ohno, S., Ando, H., Kimura, M., Ishihara, M., Miyata, S., Nakamura, S., Mizuki, N., Inoko, H., *Hum. Immunol.* 50: 47–53, 1996.

15. Mizuki, N., Yabuki, K., Ota, M., Verity, D., Katsuyama, Y., Ando, H., Onari, K., Goto, K., Imagawa, Y., Mandanat, W., Fayyad, F., Stanford, M., Ohno, S., Inoko, H.. *Hum Immunol* 62: 186–190, 2001.

16. Yazici, H., Yurdakul, S., Hamuryudan, V., *Curr. Opin. Rheumatol.* 13: 18–22, 2001

17. Gul, A., Hajeer, A.H., Worthington, J., Ollier, W.E., Silman, A.J.. *Arthritis Rheum.* 44: 2693–2696, 2001.

18. Kotter, I., Gunaydin, I., Stubiger, N., Yazici, H., Fresko, I., Zouboulis, C.C., Adler, Y., Steiert, I., Kurz, B., Wernet, D., Braun, B., Muller, C.A., *Tissue Antigens* 58: 166–170, 2001.

19. Boyer, G., Templin, D., Bowler , A., Lawrence, R.C., Heyse, S.P., Everett, D.F., Cornoni-Huntley, J.C., Goring, W.P., *J Rheumatol* 24: 500–506, 1997.

20. Mizuki, N., Ota, M., Katsuyama, Y., Yabuki, K., Ando, H., Shiina, T., Palimeris, G.D., Kaklamani, E., Ito, D., Ohno, S., Inoko, H., *Tissue Antigens* 59: 118–121, 2002.

21. Mizuki, N., Ota, M., Katsuyama, Y., Yabuki, K., Ando, H., Shiina, T., Nomura, E., Onari, K., Ohno, S., Inoko, H., *Tissue Antigens* 58: 181–184, 2001.

22. Mizuki, N., Ota, M., Katsuyama, Y., Yabuki, K., Ando, H., Yoshida, M., Onari, K., Nikbin, B., Davatchi, F., Chams, H., Ghaderi, A.A., Ohno, S., Inoko, H. *Tissue Antigens* 57: 457–462, 2001.

23. Kera, J., Mizuki, N., Ota, M., Katsuyama, Y., Pivetti-Pezzi, P., Ohno, S., Inoko, H., *Tissue Antigens* 54: 565–571, 1999.

24. Gul, A., Clin. Exp. Rheumatol. 19 (Suppl 5): 6–12, 2001.

25. Sano K, Yabuki K, Imagawa Y, Shiina T, Mizuki N, Ohno S, Kulski JK, Inoko H., *Tissue Antigens* 58:77–82, 2001.

                                        Claudia A. Müller et al.

CLAUDIA LEMMEL, HANS-GEORG RAMMENSEE AND STEFAN STEVANOVIĆ

15. Peptide Motif of HLA-B*5101 and the Linkage To Behçet's Disease

ABSTRACT

The association between disease and MHC class I and II alleles has been reported many times. In the occurrence of Behçet's Disease, the HLA-B*5101 allele seems to play a major role because this allele is expressed more frequently in Behçet's disease patients than in healthy individuals. Therefore, subtle differences in peptide specificity between the HLA-B*51 molecules should be highly relevant for research into disease etiology. Starting from the basic features of HLA-B*51-restricted peptide presentation, as elucidated several years ago, the disease-associated HLA-B*5101 was inspected more closely to define the peptide motif with a greater degree of precision for possible elucidation of disease mechanisms.

KEYWORDS: Behçet's disease; peptide motif; HLA-B51; natural HLA ligands

INTRODUCTION

Detailed information on peptide motifs of different MHC class I molecules is, among other reasons, useful for obtaining information about molecular mechanisms which could be responsible for the association between certain diseases and HLA alleles.

The association between disease and MHC class II has been reported many times, for example in the case of insulin-dependent diabetes mellitus (DR3/DR4), coeliac disease (DQ) or multiple sclerosis (DR2) [1]. The most striking link between autoimmune disease and MHC molecules is observed in some allelic products of the class I gene HLA-B*27 [2]. Another important HLA class I-associated disease is Behçet's disease [3,4]. In several populations, Behçet's disease was found to correlate strongly with the expression of HLA-B*51 [3]. At present, the B*51 group appears to comprise 27 alleles, B*5101-B*5127 [5]. Among the known B*51 alleles, HLA-B*5101 seems to be the most strongly associated one because this allele is expressed more frequently in Behçet's patients than in healthy individuals of various populations [4,6–9]. In addition, recent studies suggest that the HLA-B sequence determining HLA-B*51 is the true causative genetic factor in Behçet's disease and not specific mutations or linked genes that occur in specific individuals [10].

If HLA-B*5101 is indeed involved in the mechanisms of disease, the subtle differences in peptide specificity between the HLA molecules should be highly relevant for research into disease etiology. The basic features of HLA-B*51-restricted peptide presentation were in fact elucidated several years ago [11] and the peptide motifs of three alleles of this group, namely HLA-B*5101, -B*5102, and -B*5103 have also been determined. Due to the low sensitivity of peptide characterization techniques at that time, only very few naturally processed ligands presented by B*51 subtypes have been characterized. Nevertheless, it became evident from the peptide motifs that in contrast to the HLA-B*5102 molecule, the HLA-B*5101 molecule allows the presence of negatively charged amino acid side chains at the N-terminal position of the ligands.

In order to verify these findings and to establish a concrete peptide motif for the disease-associated HLA-B*5101, we decided to inspect the HLA-B*5101 allele more closely with the intention of defining the peptide motif more precisely and characterizing a larger number of natural ligands.

EXTRACTION OF HLA-B*5101 MOLECULES

HLA-B*5101 molecules were purified from a variant of the human EBV-transformed B-cell line LCL721 [12], which was probably hemizygous for HLA-A*0201 and HLA-B*5101 (C.A.Müller, Section for Transplantation Immunology, Tübingen). The expanded cells were lysed and the HLA-B*5101 molecules precipitated with HLA-B-specific B1.23.2 antibodies using protein-A sepharose columns. The peptide release from the HLA molecules was carried out under acidic conditions and was followed by ultrafiltration with a cut-off of 10 kDa. The resulting peptide fraction was separated by reversed-phase HPLC, and the eluted peptides fractionated and sequenced individually off-line by tandem mass spectrometry.

IDENTIFICATION OF NATURAL B*5101 LIGANDS

The mass spectrometric analyses of these HPLC fractions led to the characterization of 22 new HLA-B*5101 ligands (Table 1). We are aware of the fact that these peptides represent only about 1% or less of the entire HLA-B*5101-presented peptide repertoire, since we expect several thousand different MHC-presented peptides with an average copy number of identical MHC-peptide complexes amounting to approximately 33 [13]. The identified ligands are derived from cytosolic and nuclear proteins, which are responsible for a broad variety of functions in the cell. Interestingly, none of the ligands are derived from EBV proteins, even though the cell line used for MHC-precipitation was EBV transformed. Furthermore, the occurrence of two pairs of truncation variants of the same peptide is very remarkable (DANPYDSVKKI/ NPYDSVKKI and DPYKVYRIV/ DPYKVYRI). These two examples reflect the different processing mechanisms that the peptides can undergo in the cell: on one hand proteasomal processing, which is commonly thought to be responsible for the gener-

Table 1   HLA-B*5101 ligands presented by LCL721 as identified by mass spectrometry.

Sequence	Source	Amino acid Position
DANPYDSVKKI*	Diubiquitin	23–33
NPYDSVKKI	Diubiquitin	25–33
DPYKVYRIV	Interferon regulating factor 4	120–128
DAHIYLNHI**	Thymidylate synthase	253–261
VPFERPAVI	Zinc finger DNA-binding protein helios	258–266
DALLKFSHI	Testis enhanced gene transcript	11–19
IPYQDLPHL*	Lysophospholipase-like	24–32
NAYEYFTKI	Bak (BCL2 antagonist)	11–19
VPLDKQITI	Putative nucleotide binding protein	295–303
LPRSTVINI	Interferon inducible protein	19–27
LPNAVITRI	DNA-polymerase epsilon p17 subunit	10–18
IPYHIVNIV	Seryl-tRNA synthetase	357–365
DALRSILTI*	Methionine t-RNA synthetase	703–711
IPPHVVKV	Ras-GTPase activating protein	270–277
DPYKVYRI	Interferon regulating factor 4	120–127
DAVRIVHI	C6.A1 protein	67–74
YPFKPPKV**	Ubiquitin conjugating enzyme	60–67
YPDRVPVI	Ganglioside expression factor	25–32
YPFKPPKI	Ubiquitin conjugating enzyme E2L3	61–68
TPVRLPSI*	IRF 1	27–34
YPLLISRI	GEF-H1 protein	393–400
DAFKIWVI*	SWAP-70	114–121
LPFSPLVI	Modulator recognition factor 1	544–551

* recently published [18]; ** published in the SYFPEITHI-database

ation of the C-terminus [14], and on the other hand amino-terminal trimming within the cytosol [15] or the endoplasmic reticulum [16,17].

A REFINED HLA-B*5101 PEPTIDE MOTIF

On the basis of the new ligands, the published HLA-B*5101 motif (Table 2a) [11] could be refined (Table 2b). In general, the peptide motif of HLA-B*5101 calls mainly for peptides with eight or nine amino acids and a hydrophobic C-terminus [19]. The differences between octamer and nonamer peptide requirements are discussed in detail below. The assumption from the published motif that glycine (G) is an anchor residue in HLA-B*5101 peptides could not be confirmed because none of the new ligands possesses a glycine in position 2 and consequently, only one of at least 25 known ligands contains this amino acid in an anchor position. Thus, in the refined motif, the P2 pocket can be occupied by the small amino acids alanine and proline alone, whereas glycine was relegated to the state of being only a preferred residue in this position.

Table 2a Old HLA-B*5101 motif [11].

| | | | | Position | | | | |
Anchor residues	**1**	**2**	**3**	**4**	**5**	**6**	**7**	**8**	**9**
Anchor residues		**A**							**F**
		P							**I**
		G							
Other preferred residues	I	W	I	G	V	N	K	T	W
	L	F	L	V	T	I	Q		M
	V		M	I	G	L	R		V
	Y		F	K	A	K	E		L
	M		W	E	I	Q			
	D		Y	D	S				
			V						
			E						
			H						
			D						
			R						
			N						

Table 2b Refined HLA-B*5101 motif.

	1	**2**	**3**	**4**	Position **5**	**6**	**7**	**8**	**9**
Anchor residues		**A**							**I**
		P							**V**
Other preferred residues	D	G	Y	E	V	V		V	L
	I		L					T	
	L							K	
	Y								

Interestingly, the untypical ligand TGYLNTVTV derived from the guanine-nucleotide binding protein (GBLP, 192–200) is a dominant ligand of all three allelic products of HLA-B*5101, -B*5102, and -B*5103. This fact suggests that the characteristics of this ligand are probably not important for the incidence of Behçet's disease. In addition, the C-terminal anchor had to be adjusted. Instead of the previously published C-terminal amino acid phenylalanine (F), the hydrophobic but smaller amino acid valine (V) was found at this position whereas isoleucine (I) was verified as a dominant anchor residue. These results confirm the published data obtained by peptide binding studies [19,20]. Generally, the optimization of HLA motifs on the basis of a number of new ligands results in a differential evaluation of amino acids in non-anchor positions. It is striking that more than one-third of the ligands carry aspartic acid in the N-terminal position. This result confirms the earlier proposal that the preference for aspartic acid is in fact one of the features of HLA-B*5101-restricted peptide presentation and possibly represents the most striking difference between the peptide specificities of HLA-B*5101 and HLA-B*5102 molecules, as indicated by the ligand DAHIYLNHI derived from thymidylate synthase, which was found on HLA-B*5101 and -B*5103, but not on HLA-B*5102.

IMPROVED T-CELL EPITOPE PREDICTION FOR HLA-B*5101

The refined HLA-B*5101 motif was transformed to computer-readable matrices for T-cell epitope prediction of B*5101 octamer and nonamer peptides (Table 3a,b).

In these matrices, similarities and differences between octamer and nonamer peptide requirements become visible. The preference, as discussed earlier, for certain amino acids in anchor positions and for aspartic acid in the N-terminal position are identical in octamers and nonamers. In contrast, the octamer peptides show a preference for phenylalanine in position 3 and arginine in position 4, whereas the nonamer peptides harbour more frequently tyrosine in position 3 and valine in position 8. In addition, in octamer peptides isoleucine (I) and valine (V) are preferred in position 5, and proline (P) in positions 5 and 6, respectively.

Table 3a Matrix for the prediction of HLA-B*5101 octamer peptides.

Amino acid	One letter code	Position 1	2	3	4	5	6	7	8
Alanine	A	0	**10**	0	0	0	0	0	0
Cysteine	C	0	0	0	0	0	0	0	0
Aspartic acid	D	4	0	0	0	0	0	0	0
Glutamic acid	E	0	0	0	0	0	0	0	0
Phenylalanine	F	1	0	3	0	0	0	0	0
Glycine	G	0	6	0	1	0	0	0	0
Histidine	H	0	0	0	0	0	0	1	0
Isoleucine	I	2	0	0	0	3	0	0	**10**
Lysine	K	0	0	0	2	0	0	2	0
Leucine	L	2	0	1	1	1	1	0	6
Methionine	M	1	0	0	0	0	0	0	0
Asparagine	N	1	0	0	0	0	0	0	0
Proline	P	0	**10**	1	0	3	3	0	0
Glutamine	Q	0	0	0	0	0	0	0	0
Arginine	R	0	0	0	3	0	1	0	0
Serine	S	0	0	0	0	0	0	0	0
Threonine	T	1	0	0	1	0	0	0	0
Valine	V	1	0	1	0	3	1	2	**8**
Tryptophan	W	0	0	1	0	0	0	0	0
Undefined	X	0	0	0	0	0	0	0	0
Tyrosine	Y	2	0	1	0	0	0	0	0

Table 3b Matrix for the prediction of HLA-B*5101 nonamer peptides.

Amino acid	One letter code	Position								
		1	2	3	4	5	6	7	8	9
Alanine	A	0	**10**	0	1	0	1	0	0	0
Cysteine	C	0	0	0	0	0	0	0	0	0
Aspartic acid	D	4	0	0	1	0	0	0	0	0
Glutamic acid	E	0	0	0	2	0	0	0	0	0
Phenylalanine	F	1	0	1	0	0	1	0	0	0
Glycine	G	0	6	0	1	0	0	0	0	0
Histidine	H	0	0	0	0	0	0	0	1	0
Isoleucine	I	2	0	0	0	0	1	1	0	**10**
Lysine	K	0	0	0	1	1	0	1	2	0
Leucine	L	2	0	2	0	0	1	1	0	6
Methionine	M	1	0	0	0	1	0	0	0	0
Asparagine	N	1	0	0	0	0	1	0	0	0
Proline	P	0	**10**	1	0	0	1	0	0	0
Glutamine	Q	0	0	0	0	0	0	0	0	0
Arginine	R	0	0	0	0	0	0	1	1	0
Serine	S	0	0	0	0	1	0	0	0	0
Threonine	T	1	0	0	1	1	0	1	2	0
Valine	V	1	0	0	0	2	2	1	3	**8**
Tryptophan	W	0	0	1	0	0	0	0	0	0
Undefined	X	0	0	0	0	0	0	0	0	0
Tyrosine	Y	2	0	4	0	1	0	0	0	0

To evaluate the accuracy of epitope prediction, the probability of presentation by B*5101 molecules was determined for the newly identified HLA-B*5101 ligands and two known T-cell epitopes derived from HIV-1 reverse transcriptase. Table 4 shows the scores and the ranking of each ligand among all other octamer/nonamer peptides derived from the respective source protein.

The matrices for octamer and nonamer HLA-B*5101-restricted epitope prediction have now been implemented into the SYFPEITHI database. According to the reliability of SYFPEITHI's epitope prediction, relevant peptides are expected within the best 2% predicted, in at least 80% of all predictions (www.syfpeithi.de). The ranking of the new natural ligands and of two known T-cell epitopes with reported crystal structure [21] revealed that 100% of the ligands were within the 2% top scoring peptides. The T-cell epitopes obtained both the best rank and the highest score of all peptides predicted for the HIV polymerase. These results demonstrate the predictive power of the refined matrix. Even the ligand TGYLNTVTV with non-optimal G anchor in position 2 was predicted on rank 4 in a protein containing 317 amino acids with a score of 22 and consequently was among the best 2% predicted.

An immune response has been detected in patients suffering from Behçet's disease against the mycobacterial protein HSP65 (65 kDa heat shock protein) [22]. Therefore,

Claudia Lemmel et al.

Table 4   Epitope prediction for the newly identified B*5101-ligands and two known B*5101-restriced T-cell epitopes , calculated with the matrices now available in SYFPEITHI.

Sequence	Source	AA-Position	Prediction Score	Rank
DANPYDSVKKI*	Diubiquitin	23–33	–	–
NPYDSVKKI	Diubiquitin	25–33	32	1/165
DPYKVYRIV	Interferon regulating factor 4	120–128	30	1/451
DALLKFSHI	Testis enhanced gene transcript	11–19	29	1/237
DAHIYLNHI	Thymidylate synthase	253–261	28	1/312
VPFERPAVI	Zincfinger DNA-binding protein helios	258–266	28	1/526
IPYQDLPHL	Lysophospholipase-like	24–32	24	2/313
NAYEYFTKI	Bak (BCL2 antagonist)	11–19	32	1/211
VPLDKQITI	Putative nucleotide binding protein	295–303	28	1/560
LPRSTVINI	Interferon inducible protein	19–27	26	1/125
LPNAVITRI	DNA-polymerase epsilon p17 subunit	10–18	28	1/147
IPYHIVNIV	Seryl-tRNA synthetase	357–365	27	1/514
DALRSILTI	Methionine t-RNA synthetase	703–711	31	1/900
IPPHVVKV	Ras-GTPase activating protein	270–277	27	1/467
DPYKVYRI	Interferon regulating factor 4	120–128	30	1/451
DAVRIVHI	C6.A1 protein	67–74	33	1/291
YPFKPPKV	Ubiquitin conjugating enzyme	60–67	33	1/147
YPDRVPVI	Ganglioside expression factor	25–32	33	1/117
YPFKPPKI	Ubiquitin conjugating enzyme E2L3	61–68	35	1/154
TPVRLPSI	IRF 1	27–34	29	1/325
YPLLISRI	GEF-H1 protein	393–400	27	1/893
DAFKIWVI	SWAP-70	114–121	34	1/585
LPFSPLVI	Modulator recognition factor 1	544–551	31	1/614
TAFTIPSI**	HIV-1 reverse transcriptase	295–302	31	1/1015
LPPVVAKEI**	HIV-1 reverse transcriptase	755–763	27	2/1015

* due to the lack of a matrix for 11 aa peptides prediction is not possible ** T-cell epitopes see text

we performed a T-cell epitope prediction for this protein which could potentially lead to CTL epitopes relevant in Behçet's disease. The result of this prediction for octamer and nonamer peptides is shown in Table 5.

THE HLA-B*5101 STRUCTURE AND THE PEPTIDE MOTIF

Assuming that Behçet's disease is caused by T cells recognising a particular peptide presented by B*5101 or other Behçet's disease-associated HLA-allelic products, the peptide specificity of these alleles should help to understand the molecular mechanisms of the disease. The three-dimensional MHC-structure, especially the peptide

Table 5 T-cell epitope prediction of HLA-B*5101-presented peptides from HSP65 as a BD-associated protein. Shown are the 2% top scoring peptides.

HLA-B*5101 octamers and nonamers

Position	1	**2**	3	4	5	6	7	**8**	**9**	Score
339	I	**A**	G	R	V	A	Q	**I**		28
369	L	**A**	G	G	V	A	V	**I**		28
231	L	**P**	L	L	E	K	V	**I**		26
239	G	**A**	G	K	P	L	L	**I**		26
204	D	**P**	E	R	Q	E	A	**V**		25
19	N	**A**	L	A	D	A	V	K	**V**	26
110	N	**P**	L	G	L	K	R	G	**I**	25
21	L	**A**	D	A	V	K	V	T	**L**	24
485	L	**A**	A	G	V	A	D	P	**V**	24

binding section, can help to elucidate the subtle differences in peptide specificities of related or similar HLA-molecules.

The crystal structure of B*5101 complexed with the peptides TAFTIPSI or LPPV-VAKEI was published in the year 2000 [21] (Fig.1). These three-dimensional structures reveal P2 residues, P and A, fitted into a small B pocket surrounded by I^{66}, F^{67} and Y^7. These B pocket residues are conserved in other alleles (B*51, B*35, B*53) whereas the B pocket of B*35 and B*53 preferentially harbour P with only minor preference for other small amino acids. The relatively small F pocket, which in B*5101 accommodates the C-terminal residues I and V, is made up mainly by the bulky hydrophobic amino acids I^{80}, Y^{84}, and W^{95} which are also conserved in all B*51 alleles.

TWO ALLELE-SPECIFIC CHARACTERISTICS ARE RESPONSIBLE FOR THE SPECIFIC ASSOCIATION OF LIGANDS WITH HLA-B*5101

The HLA-B*51 alleles differ at residues 167 and 171, which are important for N-terminal interactions between peptide and MHC molecule. In HLA-B*5101 and B*5108, Y^{171}, which is conserved in most HLA class I sequences, is replaced by histidine, necessitating an alternative hydrogen bond network to the peptide N-terminal amino group, which raises the position of this residue out of the groove (Table 6).

Table 6 P1 contact side of several HLA-B*5101 alleles.

	P1 contact side									
	5	7	59	63	66	99	159	163	167	171
B*5101	M	Y	Y	N	I	Y	Y	L	W	H
B*5102	M	Y	Y	N	I	Y	Y	L	W	**Y**
B*5103	M	Y	Y	N	I	Y	Y	L	**G**	H
B*5108	M	Y	Y	N	I	Y	Y	L	W	H

This rearrangement of the hydrogen bonding network in pocket A is unique among the known HLA crystal structures and responsible among other things for a zig-zag conformation of the bound peptide. As a result of this substitution, such B*51 alleles should be more prone to having ligands with a negative charge at P1, in contrast to B*5102, which contains an aromatic Y^{171}. Thus, the combination W^{167}/H^{171} appears to be correlated with this unique MHC-peptide structure. In contrast, although HLA-B*5103 shares the preference for aspartic acid in P1 with HLA-B*5101 (due to H^{171}), the N-terminal residue of ligands is much more buried in the MHC molecule (due to the small G^{167}), resulting in a completely different recognition by T cells [23].

Affinity studies of peptides, that have been carried out by other groups suggest that the difference in peptide specificity between the HLA-B*5101, B*5102, and B*5103 alleles is minimal [20]. But as previously demonstrated, such minute differences within the A pocket have a critical influence on T cell recognition, because of confor-

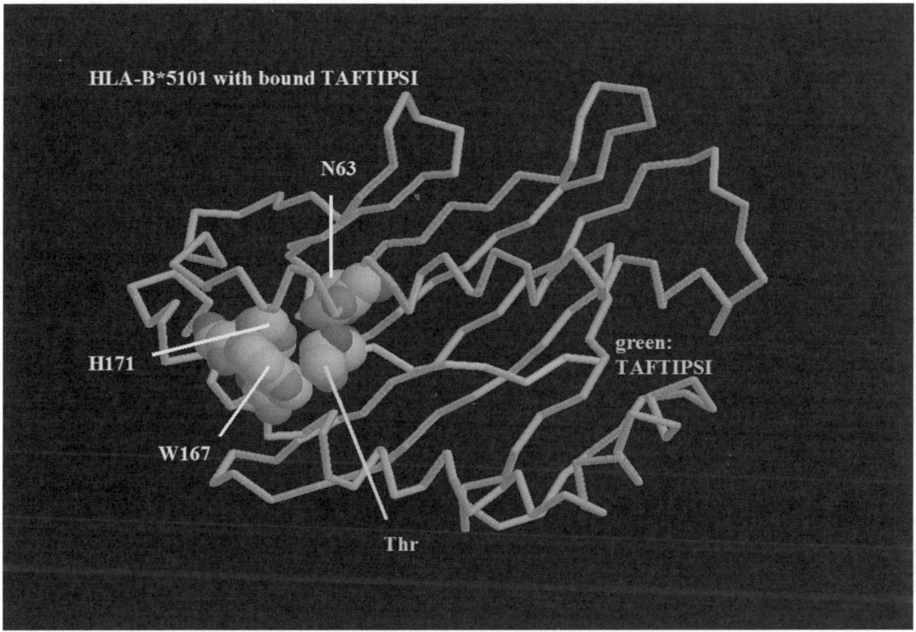

Figure 1 Different possibilities exist for the interaction between the N-terminal amino acid of the bound ligand and the residues which make up specificity pocket A of HLA-B*5101 (Structure deposited in PDB database under 1E28). The MHC molecule is shown as backbone structure (grey); only three amino acids belonging to pocket A are portrayed in the "spacefill" mode, namely N^{63} in the α_1 helix, and W^{167} and H^{171} in the α_2 helix. The orientation of the ligand TAFTIPSI is indicated as a green backbone structure, only the atoms of the N-terminal threonine are depicted by their van-der-Waals radii. From two crystal structures we know that the polar side chain of threonine is in close contact with N^{63} via a series of hydrogen bonds, while an aliphatic side chain such as that of leucine tends to point towards the hydrophobic residue W^{167}. Because of this flexibility in P1 of ligand, it seems possible that an N-terminal aspartic acid may develop a salt bridge with H^{171}. As a striking additional feature, the N-terminal amino acid of HLA-B*5101 ligands is not buried deeply within the binding cleft, but exposed far more towards the T cell receptor.

mational [24], or affinity changes of peptides [25]. In T cell experiments it was possible to prove that specific T cells could discriminate between B*5101, B*5102, and B*5103 molecules [23,26,21].

CONCLUSION: HOW MUCH DO WE KNOW ABOUT B*5101 AND BEHÇET'S DISEASE?

First, a refined and consequently reliable peptide motif of HLA-B*5101 now exists, that is consistent with results from T cell assays, binding studies, pool sequencing data and natural ligands. This refined motif enables the detection of differences between peptide specificities of HLA-B*5101 compared to other Behçet's disease-associated or non-associated HLA allelic products, as long as information on the respective HLA motifs is available. In spite of our improved knowledge about the differences in peptide presentation of HLA-B*51 subtypes, there is no formal proof that the present-ed peptide sequence alone is responsible for the association with Behçet's disease. However, it is conceivable that the preference for aspartic acid in position 1 and other peptide requirements are necessary for the occurrence of disease.

As a consequence of the reliable peptide motif, improved epitope prediction matrices have been developed. If HLA-B*5101 peptide ligands proved to be involved in the development of Behçet's disease, such matrices permit an exact epitope prediction for any suspicious protein.

On the basis of the three-dimensional structure of HLA-B*5101, the unique N-terminal binding of aspartic acid became perspicuous. Not only the preference for aspartic acid in position 1 but also the conformation of the peptide in the HLA-B*5101 groove could be elucidated by the crystal structure of HLA-B*5101 in complex with two different peptides. In this context, it seems that the lifting of the N-terminal amino acid and resulting specific peptide conformation could be responsible for the T cell recognition. In this case, could the peptide sequence, combined with a specific peptide conformation that is found only in certain HLA alleles, be responsible for epitope recognition by T cells and therefore for the development of Behçet's disease?

ACKNOWLEDGEMENTS

We thank Prof. Dr. C.A. Müller, Section for Transplantation Immunology, Tübingen for HLA typing of the LCL721 variant.

REFERENCES

1. Thorsby, E., Lundin, K.E., Ronningen, K.S., Sollid, L.M., and Vartdal, F., *Tissue Antigens,* 34: 39–49, 1989.
2. Reveille, J.D., Ball, E.J., and Khan, M.A., *Curr.Opin.Rheumatol.,* 13: 265–272, 2001.
3. Ohno, S., Ohguchi, M., Hirose, S., Matsuda, H., Wakisaka, A., and Aizawa, M., *Arch.Ophthalmol.,* 100: 1455–1458, 1982.

Claudia Lemmel et al.

4. Mizuki, N., Inoko, H., Ando, H., Nakamura, S., Kashiwase, K., Akaza, T., Fujino, Y., Masuda, K., Takiguchi, M., and Ohno, S., *Am.J.Ophthalmol.,* 116: 406–409, 1993.

5. Marsh, S.G., *Tissue Antigens,* 58: 209–210, 2001.

6. Paul, M., Klein, T., Krause, I., Molad, Y., Narinsky, R., and Weinberger, A., *Tissue Antigens,* 58: 185–186, 2001.

7. Mizuki, N., Ota, M., Katsuyama, Y., Yabuki, K., Ando, H., Yoshida, M., Onari, K., Nikbin, B., Davatchi, F., Chams, H., Ghaderi, A.A., Ohno, S., and Inoko, H., *Tissue Antigens,* 57: 457–462, 2001..

8. Kera, J., Mizuki, N., Ota, M., Katsuyama, Y., Pivetti-Pezzi, P., Ohno, S., and Inoko, H., *Tissue Antigens,* 54: 565–571, 1999.

9. Yabuki, K., Ohno, S., Mizuki, N., Ando, H., Tabbara, K.F., Goto, K., Nomura, E., Nakamura, S., Ito, N., Ota, M., Katsuyama, Y., and Inoko, H., *Tissue Antigens,* 54: 273–277, 1999.

10. Sano, K., Yabuki, K., Imagawa, Y., Shiina, T., Mizuki, N., Ohno, S., Kulski, J.K., and Inoko, H., *Tissue Antigens,* 58: 77–82, 2001.

11. Falk, K., Rotzschke, O., Takiguchi, M., Gnau, V., Stevanovic, S., Jung, G., and Rammensee, H.G., *Int.Immunol.,* 7: 223–228, 1995.

12. Steinle, A. and Schendel, D.J., *Tissue Antigens,* 44: 268–270, 1994.

13. Stevanovic, S. and Schild, H., *Semin.Immunol.,* 11: 375–384, 1999.

14. Uebel, S. and Tampe, R., *Curr.Opin.Immunol.,* 11: 203–208, 1999.

15. Stoltze, L., Schirle, M., Schwarz, G., Schroter, C., Thompson, M.W., Hersh, L.B., Kalbacher, H., Stevanovic, S., Rammensee, H.G., and Schild, H., *Nat.Immunol.,* 1: 413–418, 2000.

16. Falk, K., Rotzschke, O., and Rammensee, H.G., *Nature,* 348: 248–251, 1990.

17. Fruci, D., Niedermann, G., Butler, R.H., and van Endert, P.M., *Immunity.,* 15: 467–476, 2001.

18. Luckey, C.J., Marto, J.A., Partridge, M., Hall, E., White, F.M., Lippolis, J.D., Shabanowitz, J., Hunt, D.F., and Engelhard, V.H., *J.Immunol.,* 167: 1212–1221, 2001.

19. Sakaguchi, T., Ibe, M., Miwa, K., Yokota, S., Tanaka, K., Schonbach, C., and Takiguchi, M., *Immunogenetics,* 46: 245–248, 1997.

20. Kikuchi, A., Sakaguchi, T., Miwa, K., Takamiya, Y., Rammensee, H.G., Kaneko, Y., and Takiguchi, M., *Immunogenetics,* 43: 268–276, 1996.

21. Maenaka, K., Maenaka, T., Tomiyama, H., Takiguchi, M., Stuart, D.I., and Jones, E.Y., *J.Immunol.,* 165: 3260–3267, 2000.

22. Pervin, K., Childerstone, A., Shinnick, T., Mizushima, Y., van der, Z.R., Hasan, A., Vaughan, R., and Lehner, T., *J.Immunol.,* 151: 2273–2282, 1993.

23. Nakayama, S., Kawaguchi, G., Karaki, S., Nagao, T., Uchida, H., Kashiwase, K., Akaza, T., Nasuno, T., and Takiguchi, M., *Hum.Immunol.,* 39: 211–219, 1994.

24. Takiguchi, M., Kawaguchi, G., Sekimata, M., Hiraiwa, M., Kariyone, A., and Takamiya, Y., *Int.Immunol.,* 6: 1345–1352, 1994.

25. Colbert, R.A., Rowland-Jones, S.L., McMichael, A.J., and Frelinger, J.A., *Immunity.,* 1: 121–130, 1994.

26. Kawaguchi, G., Hildebrand, W.H., Hiraiwa, M., Karaki, S., Nagao, T., Akiyama, N., Uchida, H., Kashiwase, K., Akaza, T. and Williams, R.C., *Immunogenetics,* 37: 57–63, 1992.

*Peptide Motif of HLA-B*5101 and the Linkage To Behçet's Disease*

NOBUHISA MIZUKI, SHIGEAKI OHNO AND HIDETOSHI INOKO

16. Microsatellite Mapping of the Pathogenic Gene of Behçet's Disease

ABSTRACT

While HLA-B51 is associated with Behçet's Disease (BD), it still is unclear if the HLA-B51 itself is the pathogenic gene related to BD or some gene which is in linkage disequilibrium with HLA-B51. We have completed genomic sequencing of the entire HLA class 1 region and identified 912 microsatellites within this region. In addition the distribution of microsatellite markers among BD patients have been investigated in various countries. In the Japanese population the allele 348 of MIB was most strongly associated with BD (40% in BD patients, 12,1% in healthy Japanese). These results and the genotypic differentiation test indicate that the real pathogenic gene involved in the development of BD is pinpointed to HLA-BS1(HLA-B*51 at the DNA allele level) itself.

KEYWORDS: HLA-B51; microsatellite mapping; linkage disequilibrium; MICA-gene; MICB-gene

INTRODUCTION

Behçet's disease (BD) is a chronic inflammatory disorder with recurrent oral and genital ulcers, uveitis, vasculitis, mucocutaneous, arthritic and neurological manifestations [1]. It is a worldwide disease but is found in a higher prevalence in Japan, China, Korea and along the Silk Route to the countries of the Mediterranean [2]. Others and we have presented evidence for an HLA association with BD, and HLA-B51 was found to be the most strongly associated genetic marker in these populations [2]. Therefore, BD exhibits the same HLA association in different ethnic groups, and it is an attractive hypothesis that BD was spread in Asian and Eurasian populations from Japan to the Middle East, along with the distribution of its associated HLA allele, HLA-B51, by old nomadic or Turkish tribes via the Silk Route [2]. However, it has not yet been clarified if the HLA-B51 gene itself is the pathogenic gene related to BD or if it is some other gene in linkage disequilibrium with HLAB51. We have been performing genomic sequencing in the HLA region and founding new genes to identify the pathogenic gene of this disease.

Although the etiology and pathogenesis of BD are still uncertain, the onset of BD is believed to be triggered by the involvement of some external environment factors in individuals with a particular genetic background. Male is predominant in BD mainly in severe cases. The mean age at onset is the third decade, children are rarely affected, and few neonatal oases have been reported. In a recent study, an increased number of γδ T cells in the peripheral blood and the involved tissues, and the phenotypically distinct subset of γδ T cells at sites of inflammation were reported [3–5]. Furthermore, significant γδ T cell proliferative responses to mycobacterial 65-kDa heat shock protein (HSP) peptides and their homologous peptides derived from the human 60-kDa HSP were observed in BD patients [6,7]. Therefore, BD is probably not a simple hereditary disease and the onset of the disease might be triggered by some exogenous antigen(s) such as bacteria, virus or some microorganism.

MICROSATELLITE MAPPING OF THE BD PATHOGENIC GENE

A microsatellite generally consists of repetitive sequences of two to five bases and all eukaryotic DNA contains a family of such repetitive sequences as junk DNA. The number of repetitive sequences varies among individuals and hence microsatellites can be used as informative polymorphic markers for genetic mapping. We have recently completed genomic sequencing of the entire HLA class 1 region spanning approximately 1.8 Mb (1,800 kb) from the MICB gene to the HLA-F gene, which includes the MICA, MIOB, HLA-B and HLA-C genes, and identified 912 microsatellite repeats (STR: short tandem repeats) within this region [8–10]. In order to localize the critical region of the BD pathogenic gene, we have investigated microsatellite markers distributed around the HLA-B gene among BD patients of four different ethnic origins, Japanese, Greek, Jordan, and Italian.

Eight polymorphic microsatellite markers, C1-2-A, MICA-TM, MIB, 01-4-1, 01-2-5, 01-3-1, 02-4-4 and 03-2-11, distributed within a 1,100 kb region surrounding the HLA-B gene [11,12] (Fig. 1) were analyzed using POR and subsequent automated fragment detection by fluorescent-based technology. These markers were densely distributed at the following appropriate distance from the HLA-B gene; Cl -2-A: 147 kb centromeric, MICA-TM: 46 kb centromeric, MIB: 24 kb centromeric, 01-4-1: 6 kb centromeric, 01-2-5:62 kb telomeric, 01-3-1:111 kb telomeric, 02-4-4: 282 kb telomeric, 03-2-11:912 kb telomeric (Fig. 1).

Table 1 shows statistically significant alleles associated with BD in the Japanese population at the eight microsatellite and HLA-B loci [13,14]. All of alleles in each microsatellite marker were named on the basis of the amplified fragment size length. Among the eight microsatellite markers, allele 348 of MIB was most strongly associated with BD (PcO.00001 4). The phenotype frequency (PF) of allele 348 of MIB was distinctively high (40.0%) in the Japanese BD patients as compared to that (12.1%) in the healthy Japanese controls. Alleles 178 and 202 of 01-2-5 (178: Pc=0.00022; 202:Pc0.00089), allele 344 of MIB (Pc=0.00033), allele A6 of MICA-TM (Pc=0.0020) and allele 217 of 01-4-1 (Pc0.0030) were also increased to the remarka-

Table 1   Statistically significant alleles associated with Behçet's disease in a Japanese population (Ref. 14)

Marker	No of alleles	allele	Control (N=132)	Patient (N=95)	R.R.	χ^2	P	Pc
C1-2-A	13	240	17 [12.9%]	27 [28.4%]	2.69	8.54	0.0035	0.045
MICA-TM	5	A6	62 [47.0%]	67 [70.5%]	2.70	12.50	0.00041	0.0020
		A5.1	36 [27.3%]	7 [7.4%]	0.21	14.25	0.00016	0.00080
		A5	71 [53.8%]	40 [42.1%]	0.62	3.02	0.082	0.41
MIB	12	348	16 [12.1%]	38 [40.0%]	4.83	23.68	0.0000011	0.000014
		344	10 [7.6%]	27 [28.4%]	4.84	17.60	0.000027	0.00033
		336	40 [30.3%]	9 [9.5%]	0.24	14.16	0.00017	0.0020
C1-4-1	6	217	87 [65.9%]	82 [86.3%]	3.26	12.09	0.00051	0.0030
		225	35 [25.9%]	11 [11.6%]	0.36	7.63	0.0057	0.034
		221	48 [36.4%]	22 [23.2%]	0.53	4.52	0.033	0.20
HLA-B	25	B51	18 [13.6%]	56 [58.9%]	9.09	51.62	0.00000000000067	0.000000000017
C1-2-5	20	202	21 [15.9%]	38 [40.0%]	3.52	16.67	0.000045	0.00089
		178	1 [0.8%]	15 [15.8%]	24.56	19.05	0.000011	0.00022
C1-3-1	6	291	62 [47.0%]	57 [60.0%]	1.69	3.76	0.052	0.31
		293	31 [23.5%]	7 [7.4%]	0.26	10.30	0.0013	0.0080
		288	106 [80.3%]	66 [69.5%]	0.56	3.53	0.060	0.36
C2-4-4	13	255	22 [16.7%]	35 [36.8%]	2.92	11.96	0.00054	0.0071
		231	107 [81.1%]	60 [63.2%]	0.40	9.11	0.0025	0.033
C3-2-11	17	213	27 [20.5%]	33 [34.7%]	2.07	5.80	0.016	0.27

Alleles showing Pc values less than 0.5 are listed.   R.R.=relative risk

bly significant degree whereas allele A5.1 of MICA-TM (Pc=0.00080) and allele 336 of MIB (Pc=0.0020) were decreased to the remarkably significant degree in the patient group with the Pc values of less than 0.005. There was no associated allele in the C1-2-A, 01-3-1, 02-4-4 or 03-2-11 microsatellite markers showing the Pc values of less than 0.005. No allele at the 03-2-11 locus gave rise to the statistical significance (Pc<0.05). Notably, 56 out of 95 patients (PF=58.9%) were HLA-B51 positive as compared to 18 out of 132 controls (PF=13.6%), revealing the strongest association with BD (Pc=0.000000000017). Similar results were shown in other different populations including Greek, Italian and Jordanian (data not shown) [14, 15].

The genotypic differentiation concerned with the allelic distribution was analyzed between the patient and control groups (Table 2 and Fig. 1). Generally, genotypic distribution should be identical within the same ethnic groups. If genotypic differentiation is observed at a locus between patient and control groups, allelic distribution at its locus is supposed to be under the influence of some genetic bias. In the Japanese population, the P values were significantly low (P<0.01) at seven loci (MICA-TM, MIB, 01-4-1, HLAB, 01-2-5, 01-3-1, 02-4-4). Especially, the remarkably low P values (P<0.0001) were observed at the MICA-TM, MIB, HLA-B, and 01-2-5 loci [13,14]. Further in the Greek population, the P values were significantly low at the HLA-B locus (P=0.001080) and relatively low at 01-4-1 (P=0.00904) which is located only 6 kb centromeric to HLA-B [14]. In the Jordanian and Italian populations, only the HLA-B locus gave rise to the significantly low P value (Jordanian: P=0.00043; Italian: P=0.00691) [14,15].

Table 2 Genotypic differentiation between the normal and patient groups in Japanese, Greek, Jordanian and Italian populations (Ref. 14, 15).

Marker	Japanese (Cont.=132, BD=95) P-value ± s.e.	Greek (Cont.=52, BD=55) P-value ± s.e.	Jordan (Cont.=50, BD=49) P-value ± s.e.	Italian (Cont.=28, BD=22) P-value ± s.e.
C1-2-A	0.38152 ± 0.00065	0.10262 ± 0.00070	0.07004 ± 0.00053	0.22331 ± 0.00076
MICA-TM	0.00001 ± 0.00000	0.09689 ± 0.00121	0.07678 ± 0.00044	0.10818 ± 0.00020
MIB	0.00000 ± 0.00000	0.21318 ± 0.00219	0.06885 ± 0.00055	0.06013 ± 0.00097
C1-4-1	0.00080 ± 0.00004	0.00904 ± 0.00033	0.10165 ± 0.00046	0.07663 ± 0.00017
HLA-B	0.00007 ± 0.00001	0.00180 ± 0.00006	0.00043 ± 0.00003	0.00691 ± 0.00017
C1-2-5	0.00000 ± 0.00000	0.11846 ± 0.00176	0.07020 ± 0.00054	0.05625 ± 0.00080
C1-3-1	0.00036 ± 0.00003	0.16974 ± 0.00064	0.43685 ± 0.00102	0.20040 ± 0.00055
C2-4-4	0.00328 ± 0.00003	0.55011 ± 0.00092	0.07737 ± 0.00052	0.18600 ± 0.00063
C3-2-11	0.12252 ± 0.00078	0.61326 ± 0.00118	0.98143 ± 0.00019	0.22746 ± 0.00082

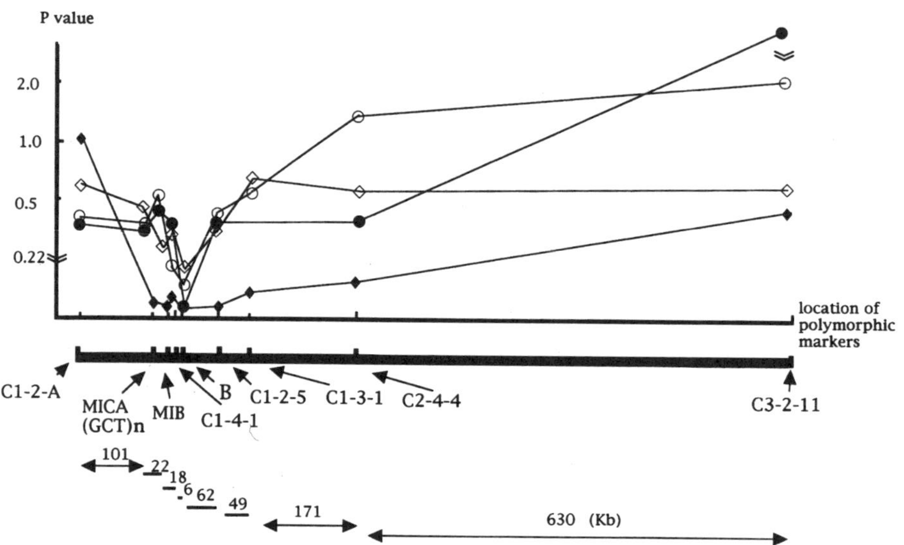

Figure 1 Genotypic differences in the Japanese, Greek, Jordanian and italian populations with respect to the location of HLA-B and microsatellite loci used for association analysis on Behçet's disease.
The location of all markers used in this study are displayed under the map along with the distribution (kb) to neighboring markers. The C1–2-A microsatellite is the most centromeric of the markers. Reciprocal of logarithmic P values obtained by genotypic differentiation testing are plotted on the vertical axis. The locations of polymorphic markers are plotted on the horizontal axis. (◆: Japanese, O: Greek, ●: Jordanian, ◇: Italian).

Nobuhisa Mizuki et al.

CONCLUSION

Taken together, distinctively significant association of HLA-B51 with BD was observed in all of these four different ethnics, even after stratification for the possible confounding effect of its nearby genetic markers closely linked to HLA-B51 [13–15]. Further, the significant P values were obtained at only the HLA-B locus by the genotypic differentiation test between the patient and control groups in all of these populations [13–15]. These results clearly indicated that the real pathogenic gene involved in the development of BD is pinpointed to HLA-BS1 (HLA-B*51 at the DNA allele level) itself. However, since HLA-BS1 is tightly linked with MICA-A6 and all of the HLA-BS1 -positive individuals in these populations also possess MICA-A6, a possibility that the MICA-A6 allele is an additional risk factor or further amplifies risk for developing BD cannot be excluded. The presence of HLA-B51-negative BD patients can be explained by the influence of other genetic factor(s) and/or of various external environmental or infectious agent(s).

REFERENCES

1. Kaklamani, V.G., Vaiopoulos, G. and Kaklamani, Ph. *Seminars in Arthritis and Rheumatism* 27:197–217, 1998.
2. Ohno, S., Ohguchi, M., Hirose, S., Matsuda, H., Wakisaka, A. and Aizawa, M. *Arch. Ophthalmol.* 100:1455–1458, 1982.
3. Suzuki, Y., Hoshi, K., Matsuda, T. and Mizushima, Y. *J. Rheumatol.* 19: 588–592, 1992.
4. Hamzaoui, K., Hamzaoui, A., Hentati, F., Kahan, A., Ayed, K. and Chabbou, A. et al. *J. Rheumatol.* 21: 2301–2306, 1994.
5. Esin, S., Gul, A., Hodara, V., Jeddi-Tehrani, M., Dilsen, N. and Konice, M. et al. *Clin. Exp. Immunol.* 107:520–527,.1997.
6. Hasan, A., Fortune, F., Wilson, A., Warr, K., Shinnick, T. and Mizushima, Y. et al. *Lancet* 347: 789–794, 1996.
7 Kaneko, S., Suzuki, N., Yamashita, N., Nagafuchi, H., Nakajima, T. and Wakisaka, S. et al. *Clin. Exp. Immunol.* 108: 204–212, 1997.
8. Mizuki, N., Ando, H., Kimura, M., Ohno, S., Miyata, S. and Yamazaki, M. et al. *Genomics* 42: 55–66, 1997.
9 Shiina, T., Tamiya, G., Oka, A., Yamagata, T., Yamagata, N. and Kikkawa, E. et al. *Genomics* 47:372–382, 1998.
10. Shiina, T., Tamiya, G., Oka, N., Takishima, N. and Inoko, H. *Immunol. Rev.* 167: 193–199, 1999.
11. Grimaldi, M.-C., Clayton, J., Pontarotti, P., Cambon-Thomsen, A. and Crouau-Roy, B. *Hum. Immunol.* 51:89–94,1996.
12. Tamiya, G., Ota, M., Katsuyama, Y., Shiina, T., Oka, A. and Makino, S. et al. *Tissue Antigens* 51: 337–346, 1998.
13 Ota, M., Mizuki, N., Katsuyama, Y., Tamiya, G., Shiina, T. and Qka, K. et al. *Am. J. Hum. Genet.* 64:1406–1410,1999.
14. Mizuki, N., Ota, M., Yabuki, K., Katsuyama, Y., Ando, H. and Palimeris, G.D. et al. *Invest. Ophthalmol. Vis. Sci.* 41:3702–3708, 2000.
15. Mizuki, N., Yabuki, K., Ota, M., Verity, D., Katsuyama, Y. and Ando, H. et al. *Hum. Immunol.* 62:186–190, 2001.

RUBENS BELFORT JR. AND CRISTINA MUCCIOLI

17. The Treatment of Behçet

ABSTRACT

Treatment of Behçet is empirical and symptomatic. The choice of the treatment depends on the patient's clinical manifestation and also to some extent to the place where the patient lives since. The different treatments are developed frequently on the known pathophysiological changes of Behçet. The objective of this chapter is to review and discuss the different available treatments for Behçet's disease. There are no evidences to support the best treatment for Behçet disease at the moment. Randomized clinical trials will be necessary to answer this question.

KEYWORDS: Retina; Vasculitis; Immunosuppression;   Uveitis; Cyclosporine, Therapy

INTRODUCTION

Treatment of Behçet is empirical and symptomatic and the natural history is only partially known. The choice of the treatment depends on the patient's clinical manifestation and also to some extent to the place where the patient lives since it is based more on the local medical culture than on scientific evidences.

The different treatments are developed frequently on the known pathophysiology changes of Behçet present in some organs.

Vascular injuries, hyperfunction of neutrophils and autoimmune responses are characteristic of Behçet's disease. Biopsies confirm the presence of vasculitis near the lesions of Behçet's diseases, including oral and genital ulcers, erythema nodosum, posterior uveitis, epididymitis, enteritis, and central nervous system lesions. The vascular injuries are superimposed on the hypercoagulability that is also characteristic of Behçet's disease and that may be due in part to activated endothelial cells and activated platelets [1].

Neutrophils from patients with Behçet's disease have increased superoxide production, enhanced chemotaxis, and excessive production of lysosomal enzymes, indicating that the neutrophils are overactive, which leads to tissue injuries. Levels of circulating tumor necrosis factor α, interleukin-1β, and interleukin-8 have been reported to be elevated; thus, these cytokines may be involved in the activation of neutrophils and the augmented cellular interactions between neutrophils and endothelial cells as a result of enhanced expression of adhesion molecules [1–3].

Lymphocyte function is abnormal in patients with Behçet's disease. However, it remains to be determined whether the autoimmune mechanism is a primary or a secondary event in the development of Behçet's disease.

Some of the many drugs used for the treatment of Behçet's disease are listed on Table 1.

The disease is often treated with different drugs according to its presentation and many drugs have been used for decades based on indirect evidences or even without them. Topical corticosteroids have been used for mucous membrane involvement, rest and analgesic for arthritis, aspirin and dypiridamol for thrombophlebitis, and colchicine for mild forms of the disease. Systemic corticosteroid therapy and cytotoxics such as chlorambucil and azathioprine or cyclosporine have been used for uveitis.

To determine the effects of available pharmacological intervention in treating the different clinical features of Behçet's syndrome a systematic review was made by Saenz et al. in 2000 [4]. Studies were eligible if they fulfilled all of the following criteria: randomized controlled trials, single or double-blind. Open studies were excluded.

To identify trials of any pharmacological intervention versus either placebo or another pharmacological intervention for the management of the Behçet's syndrome, a search in the MEDLINE database was performed, from January 1966 to January 1998 by the authors.

The reviewers processed 480 full references to identify any potentially relevant articles. All languages were included. From the 32 references included as potentially relevant, ten trials fit the inclusion criteria and were included in their review.

The 22 discarded references were excluded because they were: open studies (10 studies), follow-up studies (2), retrospective studies (2), uncontrolled (3), comments of a trial (2), patients with Behçet's syndrome included in a group with other non-

Table 1   Some of the drugs used for the treatment of Behçet's disease.

- Corticosteroids (topical/systemic)
- Azathioprine, Chlorambucil
- Cyclophosphamide, Methotrexate
- Cyclosporine
- Benzathine – Penicillin
- Interferon
- Colchicine
- Thalidomide
- Dapsone
- Pentoxifylline
- Tetracycline
- Indomethacin
- Sufasalazine
- Aspirin
- Azapropazone

Rubens Belfort Jr. and Cristina Muccioli

Behçet's patients with uveitis and it was not possible to extract individual data (1), Behçet's patients were used to validate a questionnaire for Rheumatoid Arthritis (1) and a review of the disease (1).

A total of 10 out of 32 potentially relevant references were included since they were randomized, controlled, single or double-blind trials [*Aktulga 1980* [5], *Benamour 1991* [6], BenEzra 1988 [7], *Calguneri 1996a* [8], *Davies 1988* [9], *Hamuryudan 1991*[10], *Masuda 1989* [11], *Moral 1995* [12], Ozyazgan 1992 [13], *Yacizi 1990* [14]].

Their conclusions according to the ocular aspects of the different treatments were the following:

In *Aktulga 1980* [5], there were no differences in eye improvement between colchicine vs placebo.

In *BenEzra* 1988 [7] (cyclosporine vs conventional therapy), the authors report that most of the patients on cyclosporine demonstrated better visual acuity after treatment. However, there was no difference in visual acuity after 1 month between cyclosporine and conventional therapy. After two years of receiving cyclosporine, most patients continued to show stable or better visual acuity than baseline, but there was no difference between cyclosporine and conventional therapy.

In *Masuda 1989* [11], cyclosporine resulted in significantly more improvements than colchicine in the frequency and severity of ocular attacks (p <0.001 according to the authors). Clinical symptoms were significantly better in the cyclosporine group than in colchicine.

It is important to stress that ciclosporine was not compared to steroids or cytotoxic agents but to colchicine a drug that has probably a very weak action on ocular Behçet.

In *Ozyazgan* 1992 [13], (low dose cyclosporine vs cyclophosphamide) the mean dose of cyclosporine used was 4.89 mg/kg/day during the 6 months of the masked period. Visual acuity significantly improved when compared with that observed at entry, according to the authors. However, there was no difference between cyclosporine and cyclophosphamide. This initial improvement however disappeared by the time the trial was unmasked. The visual acuity among the 8 patients continuing to use cyclosporine at the end of the 24 months remained approximately the same at the time of unmasking of the trial or at entry. No change in visual acuity among the patients using cyclophosphamide occurred at the three time points, apart from a trend to deterioration at the time of unmasking the trial when compared with that at the time of entry. Although there was a trend for fewer ocular attacks in the cyclosporine group, this did not reach statistical significance for the time intervals assessed.

In *Yacizi 1990* [14], (azathioprine vs placebo) there were two different groups: with and without previous eye involvement. In the group without previous eye involvement, 9 patients were diagnosed with eye disease during the trial, 8 of 13 receiving placebo and 1 out of 12 receiving azathioprine.

In the group with previous eye involvement, 6 out of 23 patients receiving placebo were withdrawn because of severe eye disease compared to 0 of 25 azathioprine patients. Fourteen patients had uniocular eye disease at the start of the trial, 7 receiving azathioprine and 7 placebo. In 5 in the placebo group and 0 in the azathioprine group, disease developed in the unaffected eye.

Seven patients taking placebo had 15 episodes of hypopyon uveitis as compared with one taking azathioprine who had a single episode. This reached statistical significance in the trial. High dose methylprednisolone was required by 6 patients (with 9 episodes) taking azathioprine and 10 patients (with 16 episodes) taking placebo.

With data included on the six patients withdrawn from the trial because of severe eye disease, the mean visual acuity was unchanged between the first and last visits in the azathioprine group compared to a significant deterioration in visual acuity in the placebo group. The worsening in the placebo group was also evident when data on the six patients who were withdrawn were excluded from the analysis.

In the case of eye involvement, despite the small sample size (BenEzra 1988) [7], visual acuity was maintained for those taking cyclosporine compared to worsening acuity for those receiving conventional therapy (corticoids, leukeran). These results were confirmed for cyclosporine vs colchicine by *Masuda 1989* [11]. In contrast, despite initial eye improvement in the cyclosporine group compared to cyclophosphamide in another trial (Ozyazgan 1992) [13], the difference was not sustained after 2 years. In the trial of *Yacizi 1990* [14] (azathioprine vs placebo), the patients on azathioprine with or without previous eye disease experienced significantly less eye involvement than placebo. However, the sample size was too small to generalize these results.

The results of the review published by Saenz et al. in 2000 [4] do not suggest clear advantages of some classic treatments for Behçet's syndrome such as colchicine (for eye involvement, aphtae, dermal lesions or arthritis), steroids (eye), azapropazone (arthritis) and acyclovir for aphtae. The results do suggest that cyclosporine and azathioprine are beneficial for the prevention of eye involvement, and that benzathine-penicillin helps prevent new attacks of arthritis.

In the lack of scientific evidences different "experts" based on their "clinical experience" and knowledge acquired by reading texts of others authors have established the treatment of ocular Behçet and these regimens have been repeated and changed in the different text books.

Therapeutic goals are to reduce both the severity and frequency of ocular attacks to avoid loss of vision.

Topical mydriatic agents and corticosteroid drops are given for attacks of anterior uveitis. Periocular injection of corticosteroids and or systemic administration are used for acute attacks of retinal vasculitis and diffuse uveitis. Oral corticosteroid therapy has effect on ocular attacks but it seems, not to improve the visual prognosis in many patients. Cytotoxic agents such as azathioprine, chlorambucil and cyclophosphamide or cyclosporine may help prevent ocular attacks in some of patients and should be used for many months to years [15,16].

The choice between cytotoxic agents or ciclosporine depends on the ophthalmologist as well as the individual conditions of the patient being treated, the age, sex and cost of the drugs.

Cyclosporine may be beneficial in patients with ocular lesions that have been refractory to the conventional therapies of corticosteroids and cytotoxic drugs. The efficacy of cyclosporine gradually declines and some patients may require the more dangerous associations of systemic steroids with cytotoxic drugs and ciclosporine to avoid blindness [17,18].

                                    Rubens Belfort Jr. and Cristina Muccioli

Renal impairment, hypertension, and hyperglycemia are major adverse events of treatment with cyclosporine. Bone marrow depression as well as liver and renal and teratogenic side effects are just some of the potential complications of the cytotoxic drugs. Although cyclosporine is rarely neurotoxic in patients with other diseases, it causes central nervous system symptoms indistinguishable from those of the classic neurologic lesion in some of patients with Behçet's disease and can be lethal [19].

Recent trials of interferon alfa for Behçet's disease have shown encouraging results but much more research is necessary [20,21].

An important aspect of therapy for patients with Behçet's disease is the treatment of its ophthalmic complications such as cystoid macular edema, glaucoma, retinal neovascularization, vitreous hemorrhage, and cataract since most of the blindness associated with Behçet is related to avoidable situations [22,23]. The ophthalmologist therefore must be prepared to deal with them.

Patients with retinal vasculitis are at risk of developing areas of capillary dropout with neovascularization of the optic disc and retina as well as vessels secondary occlusions. Intense antiinflammatory treatment may result in regression of neovascularization, but laser photocoagulation of the retina may be indicated also [18, 24].

As with other forms of uveitis, preoperative control of inflammation in patients with Behçet's disease is critical before vitreous-retinal surgery or cataract extraction. Topical, periocular, and oral corticosteroids are used for this purpose. Results of phacoemulsification and the implantation of acrylic intra-ocular lenses are usually excellent if the macula is still functioning and patients with quiet eyes should be operated to achieve maximum vision and also to allow proper exam of the macula and optic nerve [19,25] .

Vitreous hemorrhage is a common complication of the severe retinal disease observed in patients with Behçet's disease and many may require a pars plana vitrectomy with endolaser and retinal detachment surgery.

Management of complications should include also psychological support and psychiatric treatment, and physical rehabilitation to help the patients to deal with the disease and the visual morbidity.

CONCLUSION

There are no evidences to support the best treatment for Behçet's disease at the moment. Randomized clinical trials will be necessary to answer this question.

REFERENCES

1. Sakane, T., Takeno, M., Suzuki, N., and Inaba G., *N. Engl. J. Med.* 341:1284–91.
2. Sakane, T. *Int. Rev. Immunol.* 14:89–96, 1997.
3. Ehrlich, G.E., *In.t Rev. Immunol.* 14:81–8, 1997.
4. Saenz, A., Ausejo, M., Shea, B., Wells, G., Welch, V., and Tugwell P., Pharmacotherapy for Behçet's syndrome (Cochrane Review). In: The Cochrane Library, Issue 3, 2000. Oxford: Update Software.

5. Aktulga, E., Altac, M., Muftuoglu, A., Ozyazgan, Y., Pazarli, H., Tuzun, Y. et al, *Haematologica* (Pavia) 65:399–402, 1980.
6. Benamour, S., Bennis, R., Messoudi, M., Zaoui, A., and Amor B., *Rev. Med. Interne* 12:339–342, 1991.
7. BenEzra, D., Cohen, E., Chajek, T., Friedman, G., Pizanti, S., Courten, C. de, et al., *Transplant. Proc.* 20:136–143, 1988.
8. Calguneri, M. (a), Kiraz, S., Ertenli, I., Benekli, M, Karaarslan Y, and Celik I., *Arthritis Rheum.* 39:2062–2065, 1996.
9. Davies, U.M., Palmer, R.G., and Denman, A.M., *Br. J. Rheumatol.* 27:300–302. 1988.
10. Hamuryudan, V., Yurdakul, S., Rosenkaimer, F., and Yazici H., *Br. J. Rheumatol.* 30:395–396, 1991.
11. Masuda, K., Nakajima, A., Urayama, A., Nakae, K., Kogure, M., and Inaba G., *Lancet* 1:1093–1096, 1989.
12. Moral, F., Hamuryudan, V., Yurdakul, S., and Yacizi H., *Clin. Exp. Rheumatol.* 13:493–495, 1995.
13. Ozyazgan, Y., Yurdakul, S., Yacizi, H., Tuzun, B., Iscimen, A., and Tuzun Y. et al., *Br. J. Ophthalmol.* 76:241–243, 1992.
14. Yacizi, H., Pazarli, H., Barnes, C.G., Tuzun, Y., Ozyazgan, Y., and Silman A, et al., *N. Engl. J. Med.* 322:281–285, 1990.
15. Nussenblatt, R.B., *Int. Rev. Immunol.* 14:67–79, 1997.
16. Nussenblatt, R.B. and Palestine A.G., Uveitis – Fundamentals and Clinical Practice. Year Book Medical Publishers, Inc., Chicago, 1989.
17. Belfort, Jr R., Couto, C.A., and Martinez Castro F., Uveitis – Sinopsis Diagnostica y Terapeutica, Ciba Vision Ophthalmics Latinoamerica, México, 1997.
18. Mochisuki, M., Akduman, L. and Nussenblatt R.B., in: Pepose, J.S., Holland, G.N. and Wilhelmus K.R., Ocular Infection & Immunity. St Louis: C.V. Mosby Co. 1996, 663–75.
19. Muccioli, C. and Belfort Jr. R., *Int. Ophthalmol. Clin.* 40: 163–73, 2000.
20. Kotake, S., Hiagashi, K., Yoshikawa, K., Sasamoto, Y., Okamoto, T. and Matsuda H., *Ophthalmology* 106:586–9, 1999.
21. O'Duffy, J.D., Calamia, K. and Cohen S., et al., *J. Rheumatol.* 25:1938–44, 1998.
22. Zouboulis, C.C. and Orfanos C.E., *Arch. Dermatol.* 134:1010–6, 1998.
23. Graham, E.M., Stanford, M.R. and Shilling J.S. et al., *Br. J. Ophthalmol.* 71:826–833, 1987.
24. Atmaca L., *Ophthalmic Surg.* 21:571–576, 1990.
25. Belfort Jr., R. and Nussenblatt R.B., *Int. Ophthalmol. Clinics* 30: 314–317, 1990.

   Rubens Belfort Jr. and Cristina Muccioli

18. The Efficacy of Anti-TNF-Alpha Antibody in the Treatment of Uveitis Patients with Behçet's Disease

ABSTRACT

Ictal uveoretinitis, a major ophthalmic symptom in Behçet's disease, causes macular degeneration, retinochoroidal atrophy, optic atrophy, and other lesions that can result in blindness in many sufferers of the disease. As such, this uveitis activity has been shown to have a correlation with TNF-alpha production, and the anti-TNF-alpha antibody has drawn attention as a new therapy. In the previously conducted early phase II clinical study, seizures of uveitis were remitted by administration of this antibody, with subjective ophthalmic symptoms, such as blurred vision, and general symptoms, such as stomatitis, ameliorated remarkably. Although further investigation is necessary to cope with such issues as action persistency and adverse reactions in long-term administration, this antibody is expected to be effective in severely affected patients who do not respond to conventional therapies.

KEYWORDS: Uveitis; cytokine; therapy; TNF-alpha; anti-TNF-alpha antibody

INTRODUCTION

Behçet's disease is an intractable disease characterized by four major symptoms, i.e., oral mucosal aphthous ulcers, genital ulcers, ophthalmic symptoms, and dermal symptoms. It follows a chronic course with a variety of acute inflammations developing repeatedly in the nerves, intestine, blood vessels, and other organs and tissues. Ophthalmic symptoms are observed in about 70% of patients with this disease and are divided into the iridocyclitis type and the uveoretinitis type, the latter accounting for a higher percentage. These symptoms are binocular in 90% of the patients. Typically, chronic inflammation is accompanied by ictal aggravations of inflammation, but these seizures are remitted gradually over 2 to 3 weeks. In seizures of the uveoretinitis type, hemorrhage and ischemic changes due to angiitis, and white exudates due to lymphocyte infiltration are seen in the fundus. If the treatment described below fails and these seizures occur repeatedly, macular degeneration, retinochoroidal atrophy, optic atrophy, and other lesions develop, which can result in blindness in sufferers of the disease.

TREATMENT OF UVEITIS

Uveitis of the iridocyclitis type is usually treated with steroid eyedrops. Severely affected patients with uveitis of the uveoretinitis type undergo topical therapies and receive oral drugs, such as colchicine, steroids and cyclosporin. Having a reducing effect on the frequency of seizures of uveitis by its preventive action on polynuclear leukocyte migration, colchicine is effective in some patients but not in others. Although oral steroids are useful in short-term use to treat such seizures, their long-term administration unavoidably causes various adverse reactions during the long course of active Behçet's disease for several to several scores of years. In addition, a report is available stating that the prognosis for visual acuity was worsened by their long-term administration in Japan. Cyclosporin, an immunosuppressant, is approved for prescription for Behçet's disease with uveoretinitis, covered by Japan's health insurance system, and is used in cases where colchicine or steroid treatment fails. It should be noted, however, that there are not a few patients in whom inflammation cannot be controlled even using cyclosporin.

BEHÇET'S DISEASE AND TNF-ALPHA

Behçet's disease was previously believed to develop as a result of neutrophil abnormality since neutrophils assemble to produce hyperoxide and cause tissue damage at inflammatory sites in this disease. Recently, however, activation of T cells was found to precede such neutrophil mobilization; cyclosporin, an IL-2 production inhibitor, has become used to treat the disease with confirmed efficacy. Even treatment with cyclosporin fails to control uveitis activity in some patients. Regarding the involvement of TNF-alpha in Behçet's disease, a number of studies have been conducted since Akoglu [1] and Hamzaoui [2] presented first relevant reports in 1990. As for correlation of the activity of the disease and TNF-alpha, various opinions have been expressed by different authors with different interpretations of the activity. Sayinalp et al. [3] reported that no difference was observed between two groups of patients divided according to the number of major symptoms observed. We analyzed various cases according to uveitis activity, and reported that patients with active uveitis had significantly increased TNF-alpha production in vitro, in comparison with patients with non-active uveitis and normal controls [4]. It is believed that there is a correlation between ophthalmic symptom activity and TNF-alpha.

We also reported that in experimental autoimmune uveoretinitis (EAU), an animal model of human uveitis, susceptibility of uveitis is associated with variation of the TNF-alpha production [5], and that in a rat model, inflammation develops around 10 days after immunization with a retina-derived antigen, with the TNF-alpha level rising in parallel to this inflammation [6]. Bearing in mind that these results suggested

                    Satoshi Nakamura and Shigeaki Ohno

efficacy of the anti-TNF-alpha antibody in the treatment of uveitis, we conducted a treatment experiment in which the antibody was administered for 14 consecutive days from 7 days after immunization in a rat model of uveitis. As a result, the anti-TNF-alpha antibody markedly mitigated uveitis [6].

These results from human and animal model studies suggest that the anti-TNF-alpha antibody may be useful in the treatment of Behçet's disease associated with increased uveitis activity and TNF-alpha production.

TREATMENT OF BEHÇET'S DISEASE WITH ANTI-TNF-ALPHA ANTIBODY

The present clinical study of the anti-TNF-alpha antibody in the treatment of Behçet's disease is summarized below. The antibody used was the Infliximab, human-mouse chimeric monoclonal antibody. This antibody is currently marketed under the trade name Remicade by Centocor, and has been successfully used to treat rheumatoid arthritis and Crohn's disease [7,8]. The actual settings and course of the clinical study are described below.

The subjects of the present early phase II clinical study comprised Behçet's disease patients with uveoretinitis who did not respond well to cyclosporin treatment and who were selected using the selection criteria. Regarding dosage and administration, Infliximab was administered by intravenous drip infusion at two doses of 5 mg/kg and 10 mg/kg per administration four times (Weeks 0, 2, 6, and 10). Efficacy and adverse reactions were investigated per the time schedule shown in Figure 1. At our institution, all four patients were allocated to the 5 mg/kg group. The changes over time in frequency of seizures before and after investigational new drug administration are shown in Figure 2. Seizures of uveitis were remitted by the administration, with subjective ophthalmic symptoms, such as blurred vision, and general symptoms, such as stomatitis, ameliorated remarkably. Although our results, along with those obtained from other participating institutions, are being analyzed extensively, the investigational new drug is strongly expected to be effective against uveitis in Behçet's disease. Regarding adverse reactions, no such severe cases occurred that investigational drug administration was discontinued; however, elevated titers of anti-nuclear and anti-ds-DNA antibodies were observed, calling for careful follow-up examination.

Around two months after completion of the early phase II clinical study, all subjects had recurrent seizures of uveitis. The investigational new drug is assumed to

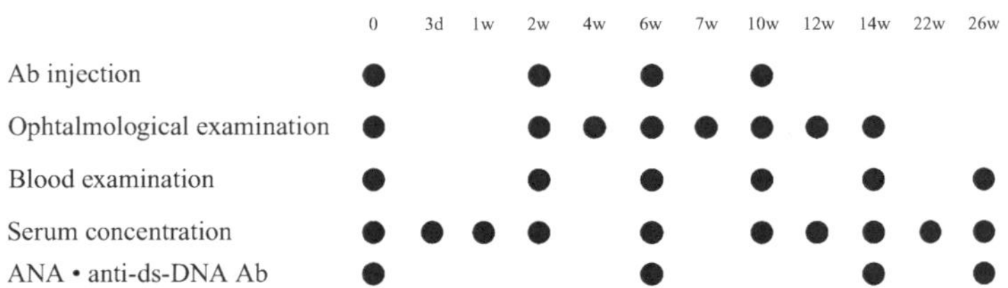

Figure 1 The time schedule of administration.
Ab: antibody, ANA: anti-nuclear antibody, ds: double strand.

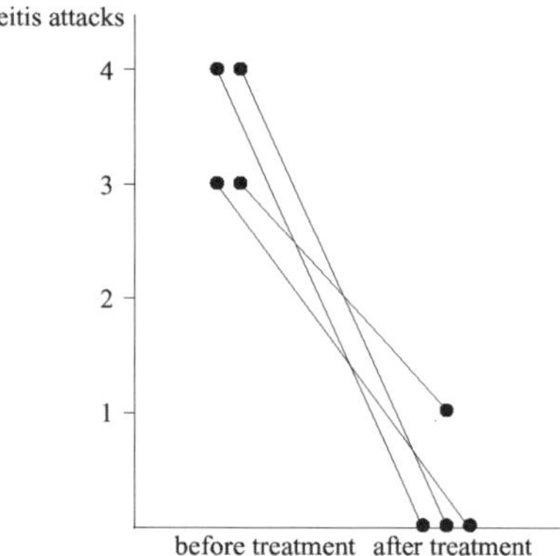

Fig. 2:   The efficacy of anti-TNF-alpha antibody
           number of uveoretinitis attacks per 3 month, N=4.

remain effective for two months, after which uveitis may relaps. With this in mind, a long-term dosing study was commenced.

CONCLUSION

Behçet's disease is an intractable disease which develops mostly in adolescence or middlescence, and which often results in blindness in sufferers due to frequently recurring seizures of uveitis. The anti-TNF-alpha antibody used in the present study is expected to be effective in severely affected patients not responding to conventional therapies, although further investigation is necessary to cope with other problems, including action persistency and adverse reactions in long-term administration.

REFERENCES

1. Akoglu, T.F. et al. TNF, soluble IL-2R and soluble CD-8 in Behçet's disease [letter]. *J. Rheumatol.* 17:1107–8, 1990.
2. Hamzaoui, K. et al. Production of TNF-alpha and IL-1 in active Behçet's disease [letter]. *J. Rheumatol.* 17:1428–9, 1990.
3. Sayinalp, N. et al. Cytokines in Behçet's disease. *J. Rheumatol.* 23:321–2, 1996.
4. Nakamura, S. et.al. Enhanced production of in vitro tumor necrosis factor-alpha in Behçet's disease. *Nippon Ganka Gakkai Zasshi.* 96:1282–5, 1992.
5. Nakamura, S. et al. The role of tumor necrosis factor-alpha in the induction of experimental autoimmune uveoretinitis in mice. *Invest. Ophthalmol. Vis. Sci.* 35: 3884–9, 1994.
6. Nakamura, S. Cell biology in endogenous uveitis. *Nippon Ganka Gakkai Zasshi* 101:975–986, 1997.
7. Elliott, M.J. et al. Repeated therapy with monoclonal antibody to tumour necrosis factor alpha (cA2) in patients with rheumatoid arthritis. *Lancet* 344:1125–7, 1994.
8. Present, D.H. et al. Infliximab for the treatment of fistulas in patients with Crohn's disease. *N. Engl. J. Med.* 340:1398–405, 1999.

                                      Satoshi Nakamura and Shigeaki Ohno

INA KÖTTER, NICOLE STÜBIGER AND MANFRED ZIERHUT

19. Use of Interferon-α in Behçet's Disease

ABSTRACT

Behçet's disease (BD) is a multisystem disorder with the histological picture of a leukocytoclastic vasculitis. It's main features are orogenital ulcerations, skin changes and an oligoarthritis, as well as anterior and posterior uveitis (mainly a retinal vasculitis) and arterial/venous thrombosis or aneurysm. Standard treatment consists of steroids and immunosuppressants. Due to the manifold symptoms and the unsatisfactory results of the above mentioned treatment, especially concerning the ocular manifestations, the disease is a challenge for every clinican.

Thus, there still is a need to further improve the therapy of BD, for example by instituting new therapeutic agents: in 1986 the cytokine interferon-α (IFN-α) was instituted in the treatment of BD. The rationale for using it was the possible viral etiology of BD and the antiviral properties of IFNα.

Up to now, a total of approximately 283 BD patients treated with interferon alpha have been reported with very promising results. Interferon alpha clearly was effective for mucocutaneous lesions, arthritis and especially in ocular inflammation with complete remission in up to 92% of BD patients.

A controlled randomised crossover study of IFN versus standard treatment should urgently be performed in order to be able to determine the significance of IFN in the treatment of BD.

KEYWORDS   Behçet's disease; multisystem disorder; retinal vasculitis; immuno-suppressive therapy; interferon alpha

Standard treatment of Behçet's Disease (BD) consists of steroids, NSAIDS, colchicine and azathioprine for mucocutaneous lesions and arthritis, thalidomide for aphthous ulcers, cyclosporin A alone or in combination with azathioprine for ocular BD and other more serious manifestations as CNS vasculitis. Cytotoxic agents such as cyclophosphamide and chlorambucil are also widely used for severe ocular or neurological BD. Benzathine penicillin and pentoxiphylline have also been described as effective drugs especially for mucocutaneous lesions [1,2].

Although there has been some improvement in the prognosis of ocular BD with the abovementioned regimens, there still is a great risk of significant loss of vision in case of ocular involvement with retinal vasculitis irrespective of the kind of immunosuppressive or cytotoxic regimen used. Additionally, the combinatory immunosuppressive regimens and the cytotoxic agents bear the longterm risk of secondary neoplasia. Thus, there still is a need to further improve the therapy of BD, for example by instituting new therapeutic agents.

Interferon is a cytokine that was discovered more than 40 years ago by Isaacs and Lindenmann, who observed that virus-infected cell cultures produced a protein that rendered cells resistant to infection by many viruses. Interferon-α belongs to the so-called type-1-interferons and can be produced by virtually all somatic cells after viral infection. By inducing the release of intracellular enzymes such as 2'5'-oligoadenylate synthetase and double-stranded RNA-dependent protein kinase, it causes degradation of viral messenger RNA and inhibits protein synthesis. IFN-α additionnally has various immunomodulatory effects: increased expression of major histocompatibility complex antigens, increased natural killer and cytotixic T cell activity, shift of the T-cell response towards a TH1-type and many more. It also has antiproliferative and antiangiogenetic properties. There are two different human recombinant α-IFN's in use for the treatment of viral hepatitis and myeloproliferative syndromes, as well as for certain solid tumours and lymphomas (IFN-α2a and IFN-α2b). They differ in one amino acid only and there probably is no great difference in their efficacy for the abovementioned disorders.

Interferon-α (2a) was instituted in 1986 in the treatment for BD by Tsambaos et al. from Patras in Greece (3). The rationale for using it was the possible viral etiology of BD and the antiviral properties of IFN-α. This group treated three patients with BD, one of whom had ocular involvement. The dosage was relatively high (9–12 Mill iU i.m./day) and the treatment period short (11–16 days). Anyhow, all symptoms (mucocutaneous, fever, thrombophlebitis and arthritis) remitted, except the ocular disease. The second successful treatment of BD with IFN-α was reported by Stadler et al., 1987 [4]. Their patient suffered from bipolar aphthae, thrombosis, fever, pustulae and "eye inflammation" (not further specified). Again with a relatively high IFN dosage (18 Mill iu/day s.c.) for 10 weeks only, the patient achieved a complete remission of all his symptoms. Later on, 21 small studies and case reports appeared in the literature [5–28]. Up to now, a total of approximately 283 patients treated with IFN-α2a or α2b for BD have been reported, 34 of whom primarily were treated for their ocular involvement (mostly posterior uveitis with retinal vasculitis).

The results in all these studies and case reports from 18 different groups and 8 countries are very promising, although it is difficult to compare them, because different inclusion criteria, treatment regimens and outcome measures were used.

IFN-α clearly is effective for mucocutaneous lesions and arthritis, with a tendency towards lower efficacy for oral aphthae than for the other manifestations. As far as ocular manifestations are concerned, the first case reports on patients with refractory severe ocular BD who were successfully treated with IFN-α appeared in 1993 and 1994, respectively [6,7].

In all four cases, the patients had retinal vasculitis and received IFN-α in addition to their (ineffective) immunosuppressive agents. All patients achieved complete remission of ocular inflammation.

Motivated by two initial cases with ocular BD who were successfully treated with IFN-α in our clinic [13,28], one with retinitis and one with retinal vasculitis and secondary Kaposi's sarcoma due to immunosuppressive therapy, a pilot study with 7 patients was performed [18]. From 1994 up to now, our group has treated 53 patients with severe ocular BD (posterior uveitis with retinal vasculitis) with IFN-α2a alone (maximum steroids 10 mg prednisolone) (3–6 Mill iU s.c. daily at the beginning, maintenance dosage 3 × 3 Mill iU/week, after 6–12 months tapering until discontinuation). The mean observation period is 26 months. 45 of the patients are observed for more than 6 months now. 86 eyes were involved. Median BD activity score and posterior uveitis score fell from 7,3 to 3,7(not significant) and from 3,7 to 0,4 (p<0,0001) respectively. Mean visual acuity significantly rose from 0,5 to 0,8 (p<0,005). 90% of the patients were responder. Time to response was 3,7 weeks for the posterior uveitis score (reduction of at least 50%). IFN could be discontinued after a mean treatment duration of 13,4 months in 36% of the patients without relapse of ocular disease for a mean period of 13,2 months [25].

Recently, a randomised controlled study on IFN-α2b plus colchicine plus benzathine penicillin versus colchicine plus benzathine penicillin alone appeared in The Lancet [19]. The authors randomised 135 patients. Sixtyfive patients received interferon. Only patients without acute ocular attacks or CNS manifestations were included. IFN was given in a dosage of 3 Mill iU / day s.c. for 6 months, whereas colchicine (1,5 mg/day) and benzathine penicillin (1,2 Mill iU i.m. every 3 weeks) were continued throughout the whole median follow-up period of 38 months in both groups. Disease manifestations occuring during the study period were additionnally treated with steroids, NSAIDS, and in case of ocular attack (posterior uveitis) with azathioprine (2–2,5 mg/kgbw) which was maintained for 18–24 months. The patients in the interferon group had significantly less ocular attacks and less loss of visual acuity than those without IFN. The other disease manifestations were also less frequent in the IFN group. Unfortunately, the kind of ocular manifestation is not clearly specified and the therapeutic agents used in addition to the study medication are probably confusing the results, for example by a possible antagonism of IFN and immunosuppressants. Anyhow, IFNα was the only agent with a positive influence on visual acuity. This study unfortunately had to be retracted from publication by the editor, due to fraud.

The side effects of IFN-α described in BD patients roughly are the same known from patients with hepatitis C or chronic myelogenous leukemia (flu-like syndrome in the first 2 weeks, reddening at the site of injection, itching, alopecia, depression, leukopenia, thyroiditis, exacerbation of psoriasis, occurrence of autoantibodies and anti-interferon-antibodies). Other side effects, imitating BD symptoms, such as retinal infiltrates (described in hepatitis C) and pathergy phenomenon (described in CML) [29,30] have not occurred in the BD patients treated with IFN-α to cure the disease by now. To the contrary, pathergy phenomenon disappeared under IFN, as did retinal infiltrates due to vasculitis (own observations).

CONCLUSION

IFNα is a promising agent in the treatment especially of severe ocular BD, where the results of the immunosuppressive regimens still are unsatisfactory. The dosage necessary to achieve optimal results probably is 3–6 Mill iU daily for 4–8 weeks, maintenance dosage 3 Mill iU 3x/week, with a treatment duration of at least 6 months before discontinuation of the drug. We would like to underline that in our hands it is not possible to discontinue azathioprine or cyclosporin A in severe ocular BD without relapse or even rebound phenomena – thus, IFN in this respect may be superior to the standard immunosuppressants. The time to response also seems to be shorter than with immunosuppressants. The mechanism of action of IFN-α in BD is still unclear and should be examined in further trials. A controlled randomised crossover study of IFN versus CSA should urgently be performed in order to be able to clearly determine the significance of IFN in the treatment of BD.

REFERENCES

1. Yazici, H., Yurdakul, S. and Hamuryudan V., *Clin. Exp. Rheumatol.* 17:145–147, 1999.
2. Sakane, T., Takeno, M., Suzuki, N. and Inaba G., *N. Engl. J. Med.* 341, 1284–1291, 1999.
3. Tsambaos, D., Eichelberg, D. and Goos M., *Arch. Dermatol. Res.* 278:335–336, 1986.
4. Stadler, R., Bratzke, B. and Orfanos CE., *Hautarzt* 38:453–460, 1987.
5. Zouboulis, C.C. and Orfanos C.E., *Arch. Dermatol.* 134:1010–1016, 1998.
6. Durand, J.M., Kaplanski, G., Telle, H., Soubeyrand, J. and Paulo F., *Arthr. Rheum.* 36:1025, 1993.
7. Feron, E.J., Rothova, A., van Hagen, P.M., Baarsma, G.S. and Suttorp-Schulten M.S.A., *Lancet* 343:1428, 1994.
8. Zouboulis, C,C,, Treudlerm R. and Orfanos C.E., *Hautarzt* 44:440–445, 1993.
9. Alpsoy, E., Yilmaz, E., Basara, E., *J. Am. Acad. Dermatol.* 31:617–619, 1994.
10. Hamuryudan, V., Moral, F., Yurdakul, S., Ma, C., Tüzün, Y., Özyazgan, Y., Direskeneli, H., Akoglu, T. and Yazici H., *J. Rheumatol.* 21:1098–1100, 1994.
11. Münke, H., Stöckmann, F. and Ramadori G., *NEJM* 332:400–401, 1995.
12. Sanchez-Roman, J., Pulido Aguilera, M.C., Castillo Palma, M.J., Ocana Medina, C., Toral Pena, A., Lopez-Checa, F. and Wichmann I., *Rev. Clin. Esp.* 196 :293–298, 1996.
13. Kötter, I., Dürk, H., Eckstein, A., Zierhut, M., Fierlbeck, G. and Saal J.G., *Clin. Exp. Rheumatol.* 14:313–315, 1996.
14. Azizerli, G., Sarica, R., Köse, A., Övül, C., Kavala, M., Kayabali, M., Erkan, F. and Kural Z., *Dermatology* 192:239–241, 1996.
15. Dündar, S., Demiroglu, H., Özcebe, O., Özdemir, O., Caliskan, S. and Eldem B., *Hematol. Rev.* 9:285–290, 1996.
16. Pivetti-Pezzi, P., Accorinti, M., Pirraglia, M.P., Priori, R. and Valesini G., *Acta Ophthalmol. Scand.* 75:720–722, 1997.
17. Lumbroso, L., Lehoang, P., Le Thi Huong, Du and Wechsler, B., in Behçet's Disease, Hamza M. (ed.), Proceedings of the seventh International Conference on Behçet's Disease, Tunis, pp 456–457, 1997.
18. Kötter, I., Eckstein, A.K., Stübiger, N. and Zierhut M., *Br. J. Ophthalmol.* 82:488–494, 1998.
19. Georgiou, S., Monastirli, A., Pasmatzi, E., Gartaganis, S., Goerz, G. and Tsambaos D., *J. Intern. Med.* 243: 367–372, 1998.

Ina Kötter et al.

20. O'Duffy, J.D., Calamia, K., Cohen, S., Goronzy, J.J., Herman, D., Jorizzo, J., Weyand, C. and Matteson E., *J. Rheumatol.* 25:1938–1944, 1998.

21. Strohal, R., Tschachler, E., Breyer, S., Uthman, A., Simonitsch, I., Tratting, S., Scheithauer, W., Stingl, G. and Kornek G.V., *Br. J. Haematol.* 103:788–790, 1998.

22. Demiroglu, H., Özcebe, O., Barista, I., Dündar, S. and Eldem B., *Lancet* 355:605–609, 2000.

23. Adler, Y.D., Krause, L., Hoffmann, F., Orfanos, C.E., Foerster, M.H. and Zouboulis, C.C., *Yonsei Med. J.* 41 (Suppl. 3) 24:10–03, 2000.

24. Hamuryudan, V., Özyazgan, Y., Fresko, I., Mat, C., Yurdakul, S. and Yazici H., *Yonsei Med. J.* 41 (Suppl. 3), 24: 10–03, 2000.

25. Kötter, I., Stübiger, N., Eckstein, A.K., Günaydin, I., Grimbacher, B., Ness, T., Peter, H.H., Kanz, L. and Zierhut M., Z. Rheumatol. 59 (Suppl 3), 50:2000.

26. Boyvat, A.., Sisman-Solak, C. and Gürler A., *Dermatology* 201:40–43, 2000.

27. Aoki, T., Tanaka, T., Akifuji, Y., Ueki, J., Nakamura, L., Nemoto, R., Ito, K., *Intern. Med.* 39:667–669, 2000.

28. Kötter, I.., Aepinus, C., Graepler, F., Gärtner, V., Eckstein, A.K., Stübiger, N., Kaskas B., Zierhut, M., Bültmann, B., Kandolf, R. and Kanz L., *Ann. Rheum. Dis.* 60:83–86, 2001.

29. Kawano, T., Shigehira, M., Uto, H., Nakama, T., Kato, J., Hayashi, K., Maruyama, T., Kuribayashi, T., Chuman, T., Futami, T. and Tsubouchi H., *Am. J. Gastroenterol.* 91:309–313, 1996.

30. Budak-Alpdogan, T., Demirçay, Z., Alpdogan, Ö., Direskeneli, H., Ergun, T., Bayik, M. and Akoglu T., *Ann. Hematol.* 74:45–48, 1997.

ANNABELLE A. OKADA

20. Type I Interferon Treatment of Experimental Autoimmune Uveoretinitis

ABSTRACT

Type I interferons (IFNs) have immunomodulatory properties that may make them useful in the treatment of autoimmune disease. Experimental autoimmune uveoretinitis (EAU) is a T cell-mediated, organ-specific autoimmune disease that can be induced by immunization of retinal antigens in susceptible strains of mice and rats, and is widely viewed as a model for uveitis in humans. When daily intramuscular injections of mouse natural IFN-α/β were given to Lewis rats immunized with interphotoreceptor retinoid-binding protein (IRBP), a 25 to 30% reduction in peak inflammation was observed both by clinical and histopathological examination. Decreased inflammation in IFN-α/β treated rats was associated with a suppression of directly measured intraocular IFN-γ levels that normally rise with the acute inflammation of EAU. The oral administration of IFN-α/β was also effective in suppressing IRBP-induced EAU inflammation. These results support continued investigation of the effect of type I IFN therapy in both experimental and clinical uveitis.

KEYWORDS: Cytokine therapy; experimental autoimmune uveoretinitis; interferon; interphotoreceptor retinoid-binding protein

INTRODUCTION

The anti-viral and anti-tumor effects of type I interferons (IFNs) have been well studied, and these agents are now used for the treatment of several types of viral infections and malignancies [1,2]. Type I IFNs also have immunomodulatory properties that may make them useful in the treatment of autoimmune disease [3]. For example, intradermal injections of recombinant IFN-β have been shown to be effective in multiple sclerosis [4]. Furthermore, intradermal injections of recombinant IFN-α have been reported to be beneficial in the treatment of the mucocutaneous lesions and arthritis [5], and intraocular inflammation [6–8] associated with Behçet's disease.

Type I IFNs, which include IFN-α, IFN-ω, IFN-β and IFN-τ (trophoblast IFN), originate from the same ancestral gene and are structurally homologous enough to utilize the same cell receptor. In contrast, the sole type II IFN, IFN-γ, shares no molecular homology to type I IFNs and utilizes a separate cell receptor. Although there are roughly 13 non-allelic genes coding for IFN-α in humans, there is only a single gene coding for IFN-β. Of all the type I IFNs, IFN-α and IFN-β share the highest degree of homology, roughly 30% in humans [9]. Both proteins are roughly 166 amino acids in length. The number of genes that code for IFN-α are slightly different in mice than in humans, although there is still only one gene for IFN-β in mice and the general structures of both IFN-α and IFN-β are the same for mice as in humans.

Although all cells are likely capable of producing IFN-α and IFN-β, most do not release measurable amounts. However, a variety of situations and/or agents can trigger production and secretion of these type I IFNs including viral and bacterial infections, Gram-negative bacterial endotoxin, streptococcal proteins, and cytokines such as interleukin (IL)-1, tumor necrosis factor (TNF) and interferon (IFN)-γ. In addition, certain cells, namely T cells and NK cells, are constitutive producers of IFN-α and IFN-β.

TYPE I INTERFERONS AND IMMUNOMODULATION

Several genes are activated in cells treated by type I IFNs, including those coding for MHC-class I and class II proteins, β-2 microglobulin, and 2–5 A synthetases. The effect on MHC proteins represent one manner in which type I IFNs modulate the immune system. Both IFN-α and IFN-β are strong inducers of class I antigens, thereby boosting the cytotoxic activity of T cells. Type I IFNs can also augment expression of class II antigens on accessory cells that in turn interact with T cells. Other type I IFN effects include enhancement of immunoglobulin secretion by B cells, activation of NK cells, and stimulation of macrophage activity [9].

INTERFERON α/β IN EXPERIMENTAL AUTOIMMUNE UVEORETINITIS

One way to examine how type I IFN therapy might be beneficial in clinical uveitis is to look at its effect in an animal models. Experimental autoimmune uveoretinitis (EAU) is a T cell-mediated, organ-specific autoimmune disease that can be induced by immunization of retinal antigens in susceptible strains of mice and rats, and is widely viewed as a model for uveitis in humans [10,11].

When daily intramuscular injections of mouse natural IFN-α/β were given to Lewis rats immunized with interphotoreceptor retinoid-binding protein (IRBP), a 25 to 30% reduction in peak inflammation was observed both by clinical and histopathological examination [12]. Decreased inflammation in IFN-α/β treated rats was associated with a suppression of directly measured intraocular IFN-γ levels that normally rise with the acute inflammation of EAU as shown in Figure 1 [13]. This result is

    Annabelle A. Okada

consistent with a suppression of the T helper type 1 (Th1) response in the eye. Previous evidence to support the role for a Th1 response in EAU includes the demonstration of IFN-γ by immunostaining techniques and reverse-transcriptase polymerase chain reaction in EAU eyes *in vivo* [14,15]. Furthermore, T cell lines that produce IFN-γ *in vitro* have been shown to have the ability to transfer EAU, but not cell lines that produce IL-4 [16]. Thus the IFN-α/β induced reduction in intraocular IFN-γ levels argues strongly for IFN-α/β being an effective suppressor of inflammation in EAU.

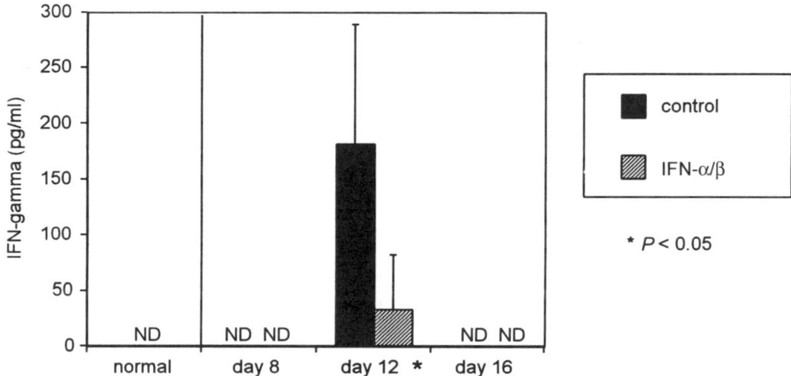

Figure 1 Lewis rats immunized with IRBP were given daily intramuscular injections from day 0 (day of immunization) to one day prior to sacrifice of either control or 10⁵ IU IFN-α/β. Mean concentrations of IFN-γ in intraocular extracts from normal healthy rats, IRBP-immunized control EAU rats and IFN-α/β treated EAU rats on days 8, 12 and 16 (right eyes) are shown (n= 5). IFN-γ detection limit = 13 pg/ml.

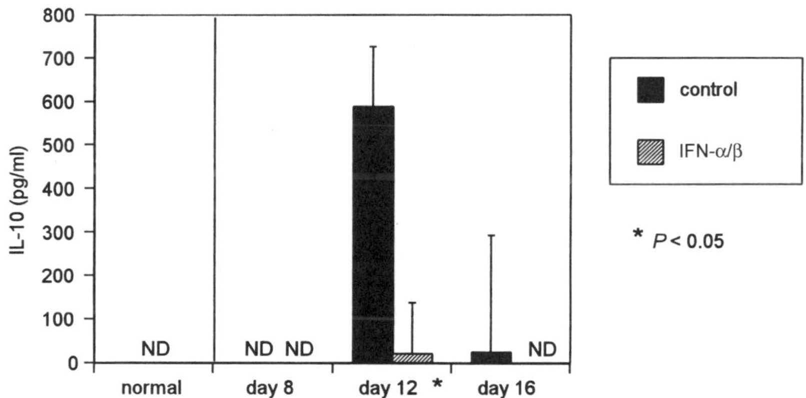

Figure 2 Lewis rats immunized with IRBP were given daily intramuscular injections from day 0 (day of immunization) to one day prior to sacrifice of either control or 10⁵ IU IFN-α/β. Mean concentrations of IFN-γ in intraocular extracts from normal healthy rats, IRBP-immunized control EAU rats and IFN-α/β treated EAU rats on days 8, 12 and 16 (right eyes) are shown (n= 5). IL-10 detection limit = 15.6 pg/ml.

Interestingly, when IRBP-immunized Lewis rats were treated with IFN-α/β, in-traocular IL-10 levels were also suppressed during peak EAU as shown in Figure 2 [13]. This result renders unlikely the possibility of local activation of a Th2 response. It may be that both intraocular Th1 and Th2 responses are co-suppressed with IFN-α/β. This would be in agreement with studies in multiple sclerosis patients, in which IFN-β was found to have no influence on numbers of IL-10 secreting Th2 cells in peripheral blood mononuclear cell cultures, and it has been tentatively suggested that IFN-β does not activate Th2 cells in these patients [4]. Furthermore, a regulatory T cell associated with transforming growth factor (TGF)-β production, capable of suppressing both Th1 and Th2 responses, may be involved in the response to IFN-α/β treatment [17, 18]. Other ways in which IFN-α/β might influence intraocular cytokine production and suppress local inflammation must also be considered, including de-creased peripheral immune cell trafficking to the eye by alteration of cell adhesion molecule expression on vascular endothelial cells.

The oral administration of type I IFN was also found to be capable of suppressing EAU in IRBP-immunized rats [19]. Spleen cell proliferation and IFN-γ production from rats treated with IFN-β were significantly decreased compared to controls. Fur-thermore, the proportion of both NK cells and NK-T cells in the peripheral blood of rats treated with IFN-β was increased compared to controls. These results suggest that the oral administration of IFN-β reduces inflammation in IRBP-mediated EAU, and that the mechanism of this action may involve NK cells and NK-T cells.

The mechanism of action of orally-administered IFN is believed to distinct from that given either intravenously or injected intradermally or intramuscularly. This is based on animal studies showing that oral administration of IFN-α in mice does not result in detectable levels of IFN-α in the serum [20]. Furthermore, in contrast to intraperitoneal administration, circulating antibody to IFN does not block the suppres-sive effect that orally-administered IFN has on peripheral white blood cell counts [21]. Moreover, it has been shown that low dose IFN, while ineffective if given parenteral-ly, is able to suppress acute experimental autoimmune encephalomyelitis when given orally [22]. Such potential efficacy, combined with the obvious benefit of ease of administration, has made oral IFN therapy a viable alternative to injected therapy. Clinically, the oral administration of type I IFN has been shown to be effective in patients with multiple sclerosis [23], rheumatoid arthritis, insulin-dependent diabetes mellitus (IDDM) [24] and Sjögren's syndrome [25].

CONCLUSION

Type I IFNs, administered either as an intramuscular injection or orally, are capable of suppressing EAU inflammation in IRBP-immunized Lewis rats. This suppressive effect is associated with a reduction in the normally elevated intraocular IFN-γ and IL-10 levels observed in EAU. Finally, these results support continued investigation of the effect of type I IFN therapy in both experimental and clinical uveitis.

REFERENCES

1. Baron, S., Tyring, S.K., Fleischmann, W.R., Coppenhaver, D.H., Niesel, D.W., Klimpel, G.R., Stanton G.J. and Hughes, T.K. *J. Am. Med. Assoc.* 266: 1375–1383, 1991.
2. Borden, E.C. *N. Engl. J. Med.* 326: 1198–1205, 1992.
3. Belardelli, F. and Gresser, I. *Immunol. Today* 17: 369–372, 1996.
4. Arnason, B.G.W. *Clin. Immunol. Immunopathol.* 81: 1–11, 1996.
5. O'Duffy, J.D., Calamia, K., Cohen, S., Goronzy, J.J., Herman, D., Jorizzo, J., Weyand, C. and Matteson, E. *J. Rheumatol.* 25: 1938–1944, 1998.
6. Feron, E.J., Rothova, A., van Hagen, P.M., Baarsma, G.S. and Suttorp-Schulten, M.S.A. Lancet 343: 1428, 1994.
7. Kötter, I., Eckstein, A.K., Stübiger, N. and Zierhut, M. *Br. J. Ophthalmol.* 82: 488–494, 1998.
8. Demiroglu, H., Ozcebe, O.I., Barista, I., Dundar, S. and Eldem, B. *Lancet* 355: 605–609, 2000.
9. De Maeyer, E. and De Maeyer-Guignard, J. in: *The Cytokine Handbook*, Thomson, A. (ed), pp. 265–288, Academic Press, London, 1994.
10. Nussenblatt, R.B., Kuwabara, R.T., Monasterio, F.M. and Wacker, W.B. *Arch. Opthalmol.* 99: 1090–1092, 1981.
11. Caspi, R.R., Roberg, F.G., Chann, C.C., Wiggert, B., Charder, G.J., Rozenszajn, L.A., Lando, Z. and Nussenblatt, R.B. (1988). *J. Immunol.* 140: 1490–1495, 1988.
12. Okada, A.A., Keino, H., Fukai, T., Sakai, J., Usui, M. and Mizuguchi, J. *Ocular Inflamm. Immunol.* 6: 215–226, 1998.
13. Okada, A.A., Keino, H., Suzuki, J., Sakai, J., Usui, M. and Mizuguchi, J. *Int. Immunol.* 10: 1917–1922, 1998.
14. Charteris, D.G. and Lightman, S.L. *Immunology* 75:463–467, 1992.
15. Barton, K., McLauchlan, M.T., Calder, V.L. and Lightman, S. *Cell. Immunol.* 164: 133–140, 1995.
16. Caspi, R.R., Sun, B., Agarwal, R.K., Silver, P.B., Rizzo, L.V., Chan, C.C., Wiggert, B. and Wilder, R.L. *Eye* 11: 209–212, 1997.
17. O'Garra, A. *Immunity* 8: 275–283, 1998.
18. Bridoux, F., Badou, A., Saoudi, A., Bernard, I., Druet, E., Pasquier, R., Druet, P. and Pelletier, L. *J. Exp. Med.* 185: 1769–1775, 1997.
19. Suzuki, J., Sakai, J., Okada, A.A., Takada, E., Usui, M. and Mizuguchi J. *Graefe's Arch. Clin. Exp. Ophthalmol.* 240:314–321, 2002.
20. Eid, P., Meritet, J.F., Maury, C., Lasfar, A., Weill, D. and Tovey, M.G. *J. Interferon Cytokine. Res.* 19: 157–169, 1999.
21. Fleischmann, W.R., Koren, S. and Fleischmann, C.M. *Proc. Soc. Exp. Biol. Med.* 201: 199–207, 1992.
22. Brod, S.A., Scott, M., Burns, D.K. and Phillips, J.T. *J. Interferon Cytokine. Res.* 15: 115–122, 1995.
23. Brod, S.A., Kerman, R.H., Nelson, L.D., Marshall, G.D., Jr., Henninger, E.M., Khan, M., Jin, R. and Wolinsky, J.S. *Mult. Scler.* 3: 1–7, 1997.
24. Brod, S. A. *J. Interferon Cytokine. Res.* 19: 841–852, 1999.
25. Ship, J.A., Fox, P.C., Michalek, J.E., Cummins, M.J. and Richards, A.B. *J. Interferon Cytokine Res.* 19, 943–951, 1999.

Authors

ADLER, YAEL

Department of Dermatology
University Hospital Benjamin Franklin
Berlin, Germany

AKBARIAN, MAHMOOD

Behçet's Disease Unit
Rheumatology Research Center
Shariati Hospital
Teheran University for Medical Sciences
Teheran, Iran

BANG, DONGSINK

Department of Dermatology
Yonsei University College of Medicine
Seoul, Korea

BELFORT, RUBENS JR.

Department of Ophthalmology
Federal University of São Paulo
São Paulo, Brazil

BRAUN, BEATE

Department Internal Medicine II and
Section of Transplantation Immunology and
Immunohematology
University of Tuebingen
Tuebingen, Germany

CHAMS, CHEYDA

Behçet's Disease Unit
Rheumatology Research Center
Shariati Hospital
Teheran University for Medical Science
Teheran, Iran

CHAMS, HORMOZ

Behçet's Disease Unit
Rheumatology Research Center
Shariati Hospital
Teheran University for Medical Science
Teheran, Iran

DAVATCHI, FEREYDOUN

Behçet's Disease Unit
Rheumatology Research Center
Shariati Hospital
Teheran University for Medical Sciences
Teheran, Iran

FRESKO, IZZET

Department of Medicine
Cerraphasa Medical School
Istanbul, Turkey

GHARIBDOOST, FARHAD

Behçet's Disease Unit
Rheumatology Research Center
Shariati Hospital
Teheran University for Medical Science
Teheran, Iran

GÜL, AHMET

Division of Rheumatology
Department of Internal Medicine
Faculty of Medicine
University of Istanbul
Istanbul, Turkey

GÜNAYDIN, ILHAN

Department Internal Medicine II
University of Tuebingen
Tuebingen, Germany

INOKO, HIDETOSHI

Department of Genetic Information
Division of Molecular Life Science
Tokai University School of Medicine
Bohseidai
Isehara, Japan

IWABUCHI, CHIKAKO

Division of Immunobiology,
Institute for Genetic Medicine
Hokkaido University
Sapporo, Japan

IWABUCHI, KAZUYA

Division of Immunobiology
Institute for Genetic Medicine
Hokkaido University
Sapporo, Japan

JAMSHIDI, AHMAD-REZA

Behçet's Disease Unit
Rheumatology Research Center
Shariati Hospital
Teheran University for Medical Science
Teheran, Iran

KAISER, ELIZABETH D.E.

Doheny Eye Institute
University of Southern California
School of Medicine
Los Angeles, CA, USA

KIMURA, MINORU

Department of Molecular Life Science
Institute of Medical Sciences, Bohseidai
Isehara, Japan

KIMURA, TAKAHIRO

Department of Molecular Life Science
School of Medicine, Bohseidai
Isehara, Japan

KITAICHI, NOBUYOSHI

Department of Ophthalmology
Graduate School of Medicine
Hokkaido University
Sapporo, Japan

KÖTTER, INA

Department Internal Medicine II
University of Tuebingen
Tuebingen, Germany

KURZ, BERND

Department Internal Medicine II
Section of Transplantation Immunology and
Immunohematology
University of Tuebingen
Tuebingen, Germany

LEE, EUN-SO

Department of Dermatology
Ajou University School of Medicine
Suwon, Korea

LEE, SUNGNACK

Department of Dermatology
Ajou University School of Medicine
Suwon, Korea

LEHNER, THOMAS

Peter Gorer Department of Immunobiology
Guy's, King's & St Thomas' School of
Medicine
Guy's Hospital
London, England

LEMMEL, CLAUDIA

Institute of Cell Biology
Department of Immunology
University of Tuebingen
Tuebingen, Germany

MIZUKI, NOBUHISA

Department of Ophthalmology
Yokohama City University
School of Medicine
Yokohama, Japan

MUCCIOLI, CRISTINA

Department of Ophthalmology
Federal University of São Paulo
São Paulo, Brazil

MÜLLER, CLAUDIA A.

Department Internal Medicine II and
Section of Transplantation Immunology and
Immunohematology
University of Tuebingen
Tuebingen, Germany

NADJI, ABDOL-HADI

Behçet's Disease Unit
Rheumatology Research Center
Shariati Hospital
Teheran University for Medical Sciences
Teheran, Iran

NAGAFUCHI, HIROKO

Departments of Immunology and Medicine,
and Institute of Medical Science
St. Marianna University School of Medicine
Kawasaki, Japan

NAKAMURA, SATOSHI

Department of Ophthalmology
Yokohama City University
School of Medicine
Yokohama, Japan

NISHIDA, TOMOMI

Department of Ophthalmology
Yokohama City University
School of Medicine
Yokohama, Japan

NOMURA, EI-ICHI

Department of Molecular Life Science
School of Medicine, Bohseidai
Isehara, Japan

OHNO, SHIGEAKI

Department of Ophthalmology and
Visual Sciences
Hokkaido University
Graduate School of Medicine
Sapporo, Japan

OKADA, ANNABELLE A.

Department of Ophthalmology
Kyorin University School of Medicine
Mitaka
Tokyo, Japan

ONOÉ, KAZUNORI

Division of Immunobiology
Institute for Genetic Medicine
Hokkaido University
Sapporo, Japan

OZYAZGAN, YILMAZ — Cerrahpasa Medical Faculty
Hospital Istanbul University
Istanbul, Turkey

RAMMENSEE, HANS-GEORG — Institute for Cell Biology
Department of Immunology
University of Tuebingen
Tuebingen, Germany

RAO, NARSING A. — Uveitis Service and A. Ray Irvine Ophthalmic
Pathology Laboratory
Doheny Eye Institute
Los Angeles, CA, USA

SAKANE, TSUYOSHI — Departments of Immunology and Medicine,
St. Marianna University School of Medicine
Kawasaki, Japan

SATO, MASAHIRO — The Institute of Medical Sciences, Bohseidai
Isehara, Japan

SHAHRAM, FARHAD — Behçet's Disease Unit
Rheumatology Research Center
Shariati Hospital, Teheran
University for Medical Sciences
Teheran, Iran

SHIMOYAMA, YOSHIHIRO — Departments of Immunology and Medicine,
St. Marianna University School of Medicine
Kawasaki, Japan

SOHN, SEONGHYANG — Laboratory of Cell Biology
Ajou University Institute for Medical Science
Suwon, Korea

STEIERT, INGE — Department Internal Medicine II and
Section of Transplantation Immunology and
Immunohematology
University of Tuebingen
Tuebingen, Germany

STEVANOVIČ, STEFAN — Institute for Cell Biology
Department of Immunology
University of Tuebingen
Tuebingen, Germany

STÜBIGER, NICOLE — Department of Ophthalmology I
University of Tuebingen
Tuebingen, Germany

SUZUKI, NOBORU

Departments of Immunology and Medicine,
St. Marianna University School of Medicine
Kawasaki, Japan

TAKEBA, YUKO

Departments of Immunology and Medicine,
St. Marianna University School of Medicine
Kawasaki, Japan

TAKENO, MITSUHIRO

Departments of Immunology and Medicine,
St. Marianna University School of Medicine
Kawasaki, Japan

WATANABE, TOSHITERU

Institute of Medical Sciences, Bohseidai
Isehara, Japan

WERNET, DOROTHEE

Department of Transfusion Medicine
University of Tuebingen
Tuebingen, Germany

YAZICI, HASAN

Cerrahpasa Medical Faculty
Hospital Istanbul University
Istanbul, Turkey

ZIERHUT, MANFRED

Department of Ophthalmology I
University of Tuebingen
Tuebingen, Germany

ZOUBOULIS, CHRISTOS C.

Department of Dermatology
University Hospital Benjamin Franklin
Berlin, Germany

Index